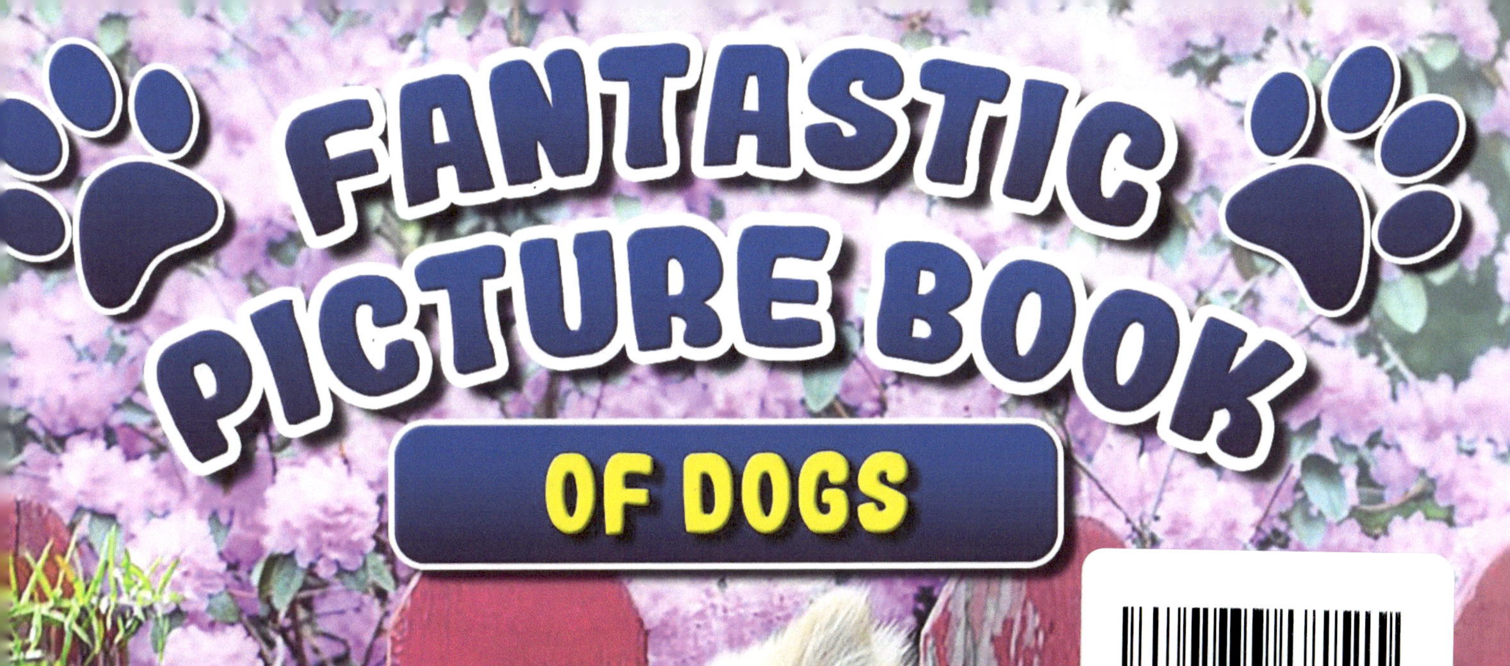

Copyright © Rodrick Madison

All rights reserved. This book or any portion thereof may not be reproduced or used in any manner whatsoever without the express written permission of the publisher except for the use of brief quotations in a book review.

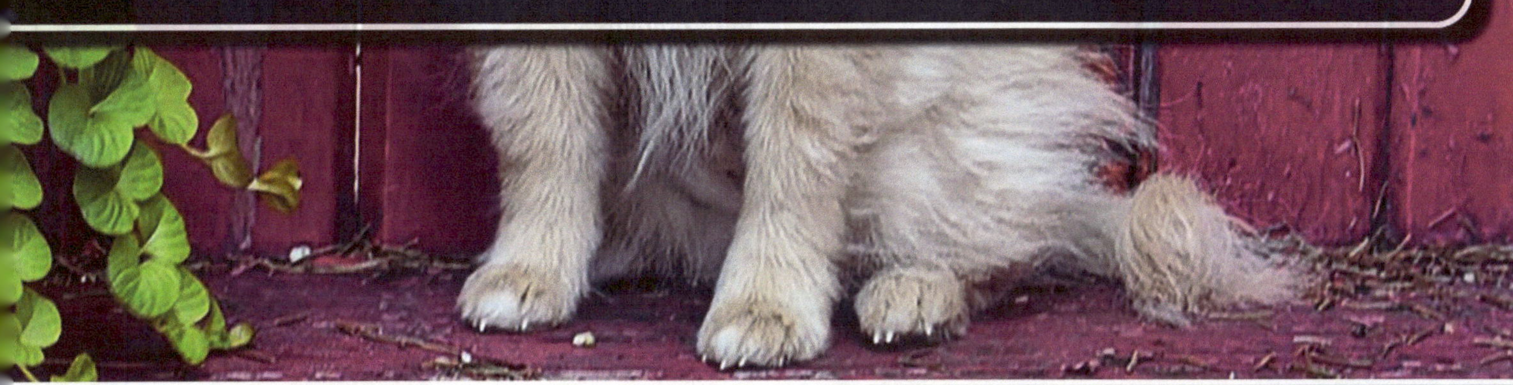

AFGHAN HOUND

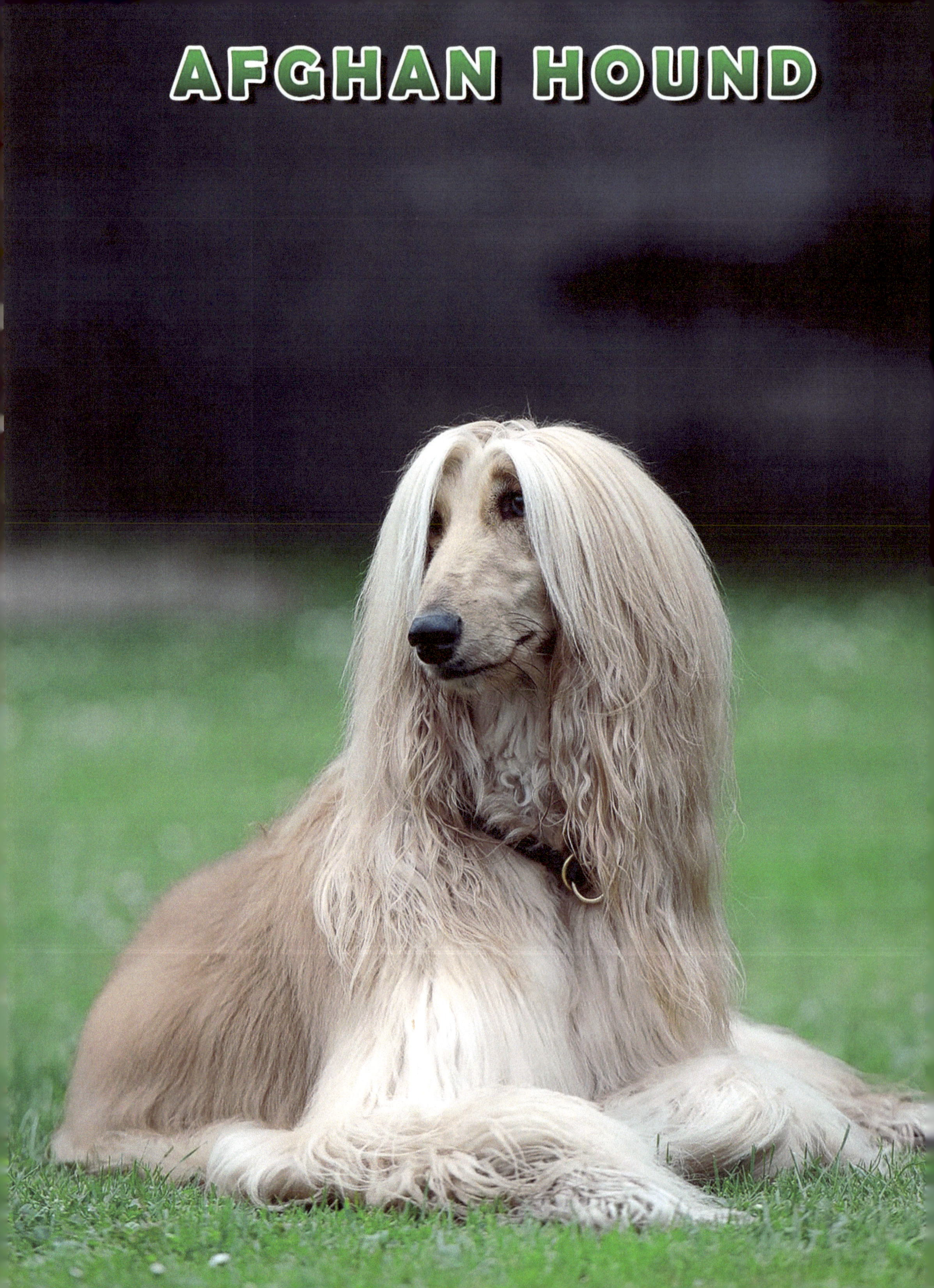

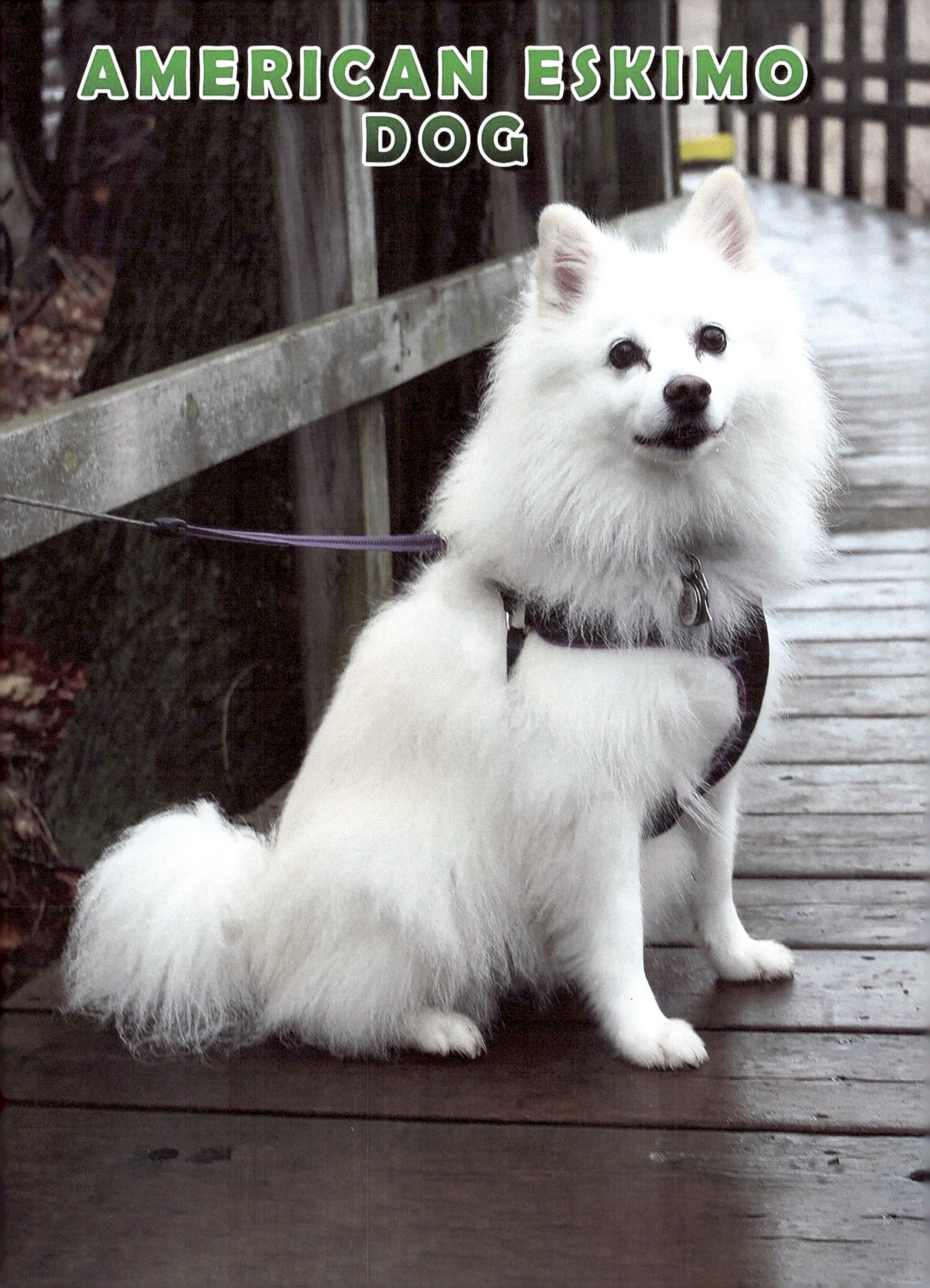

AMERICAN ESKIMO DOG

AMERICAN PIT BULL TERRIER

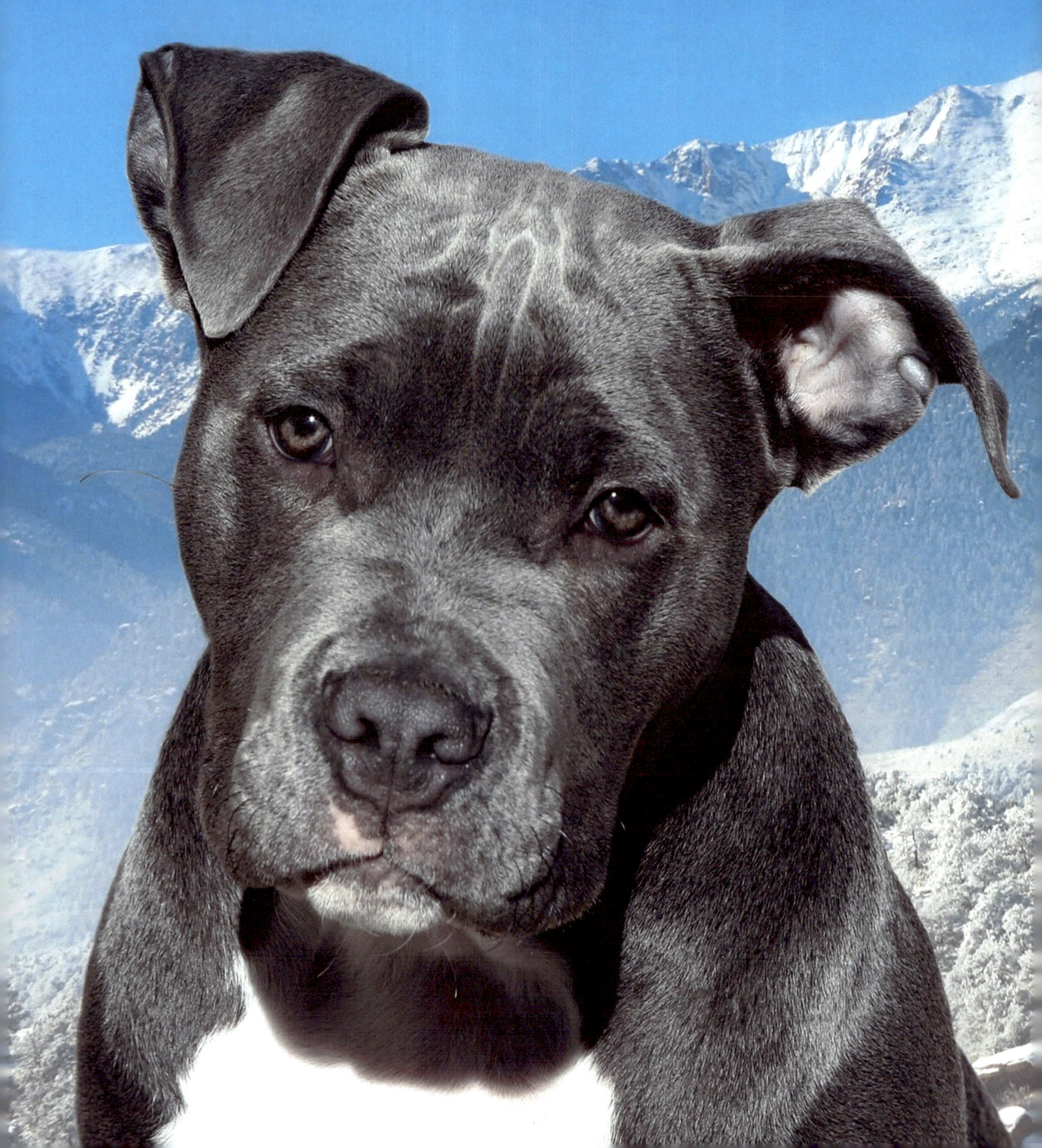

AUSTRALIAN SHEPHERD

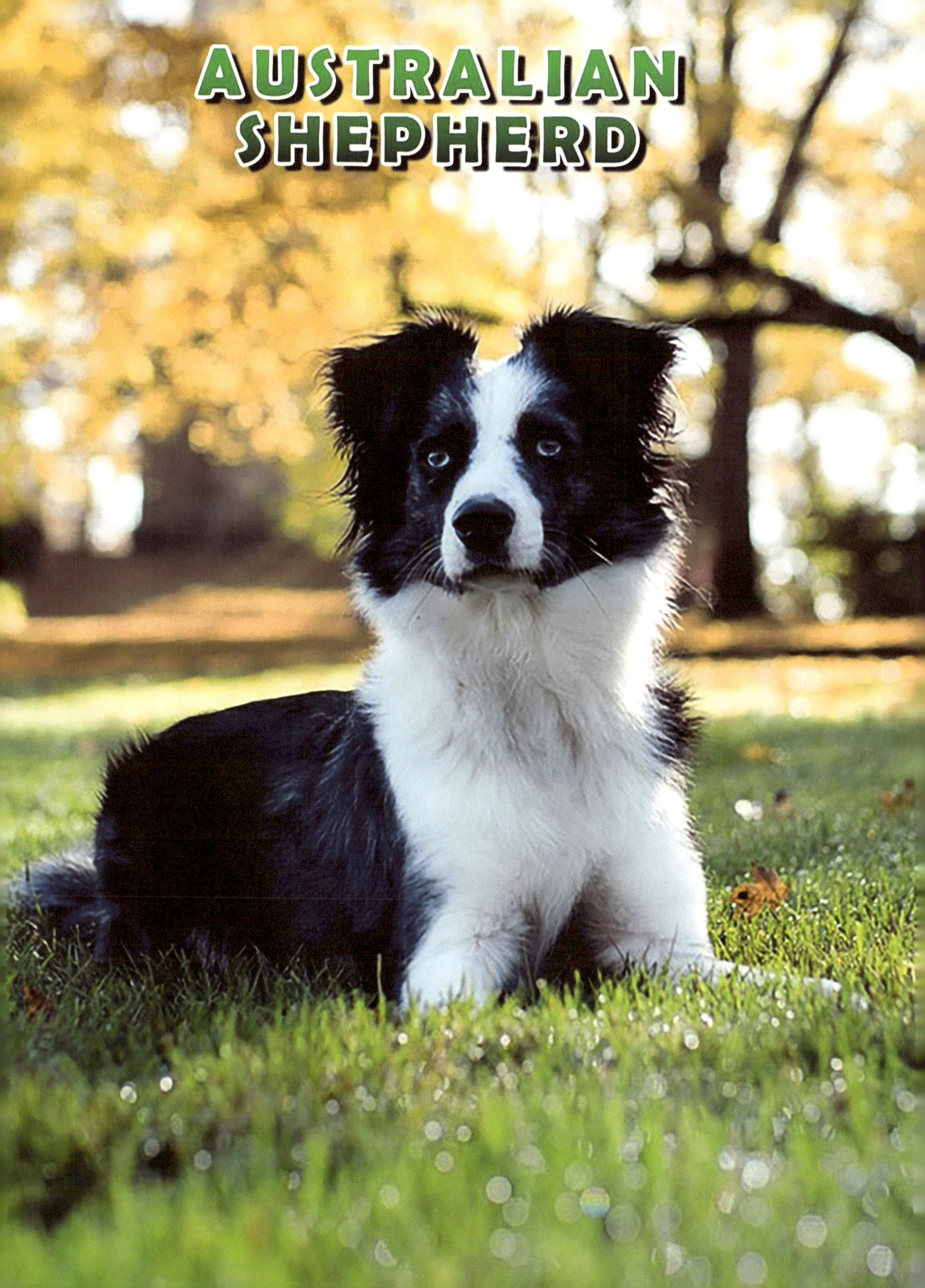

BASENJI

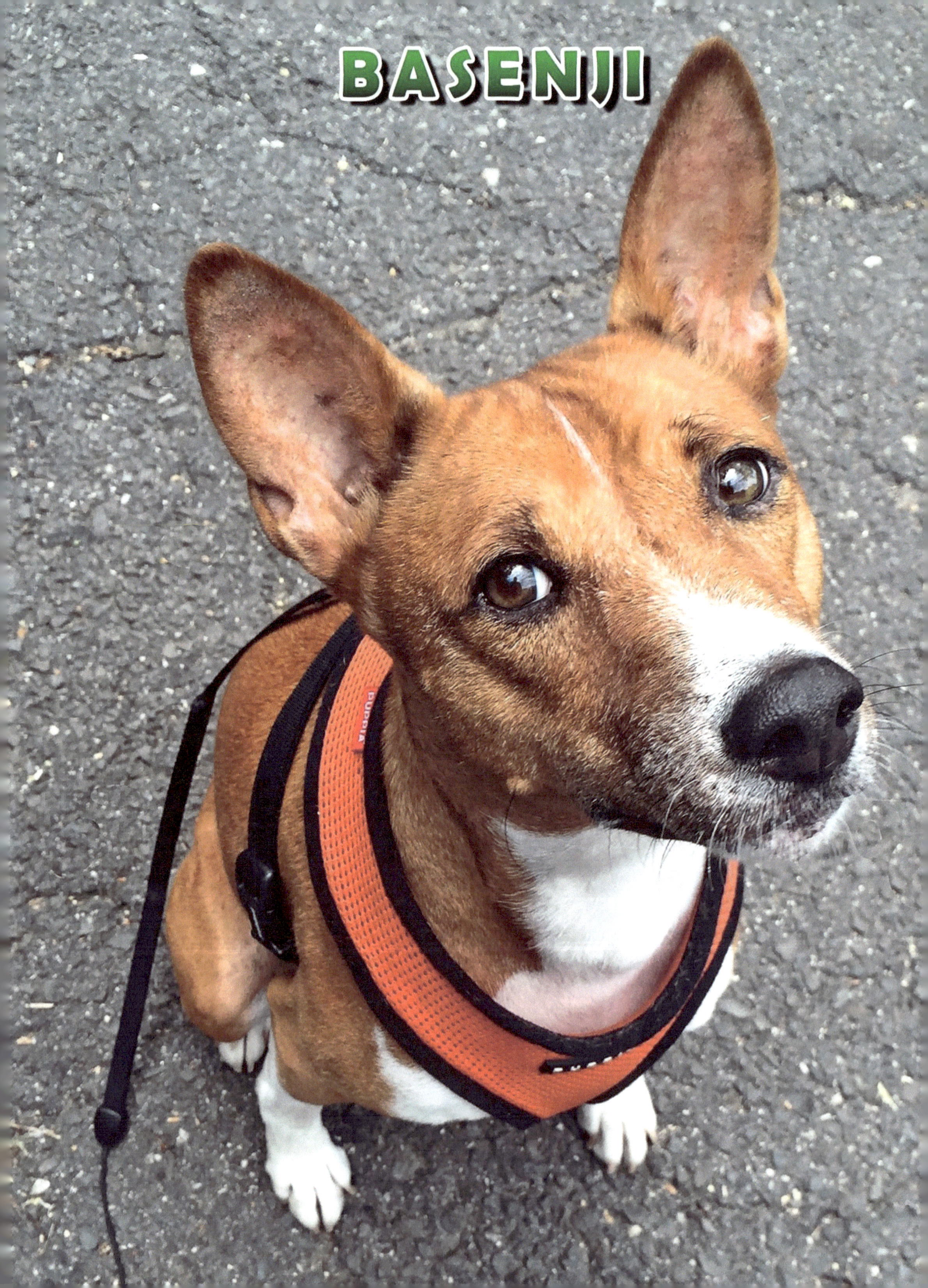

BASSET HOUND

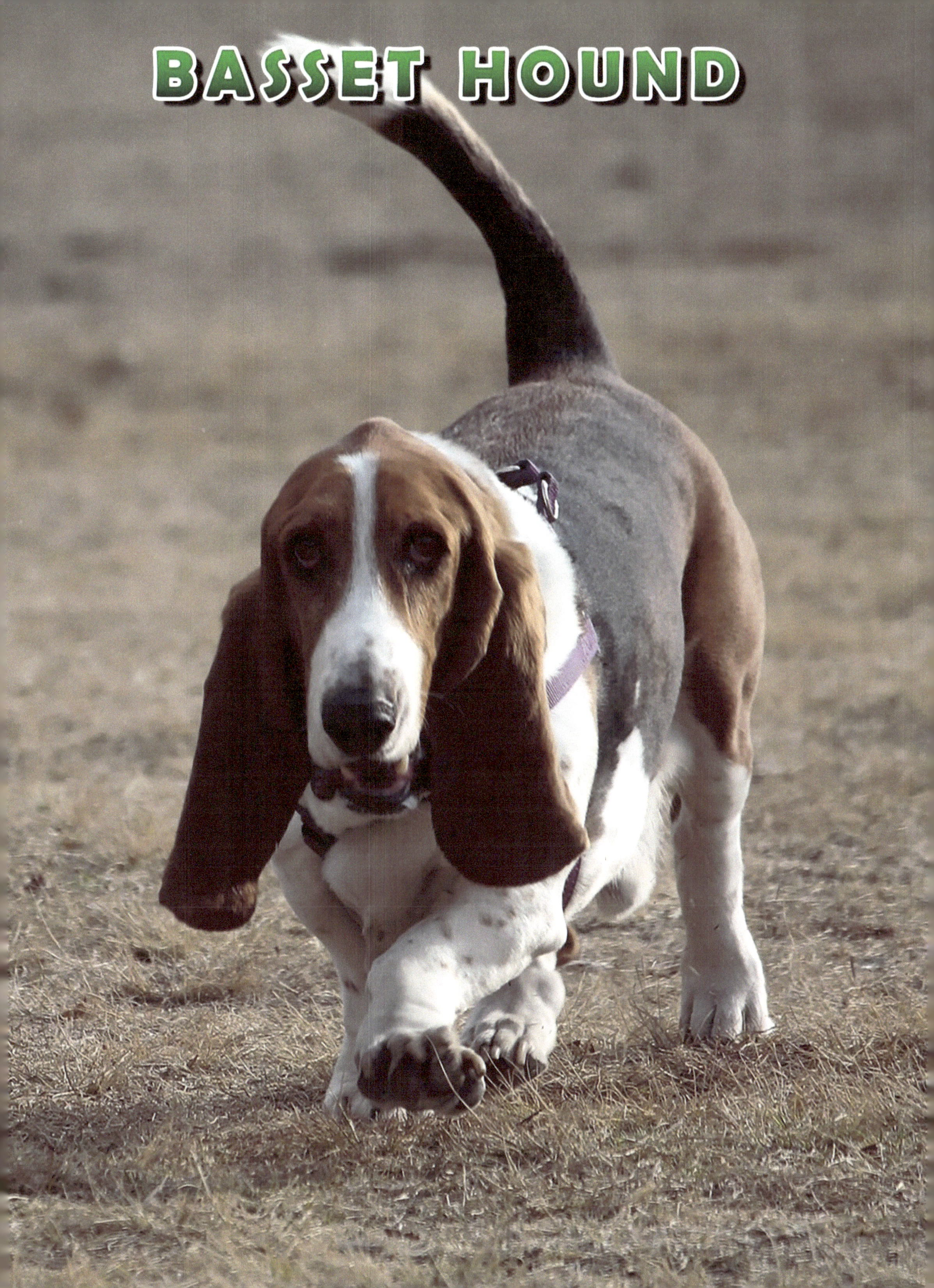

BEAUCERON

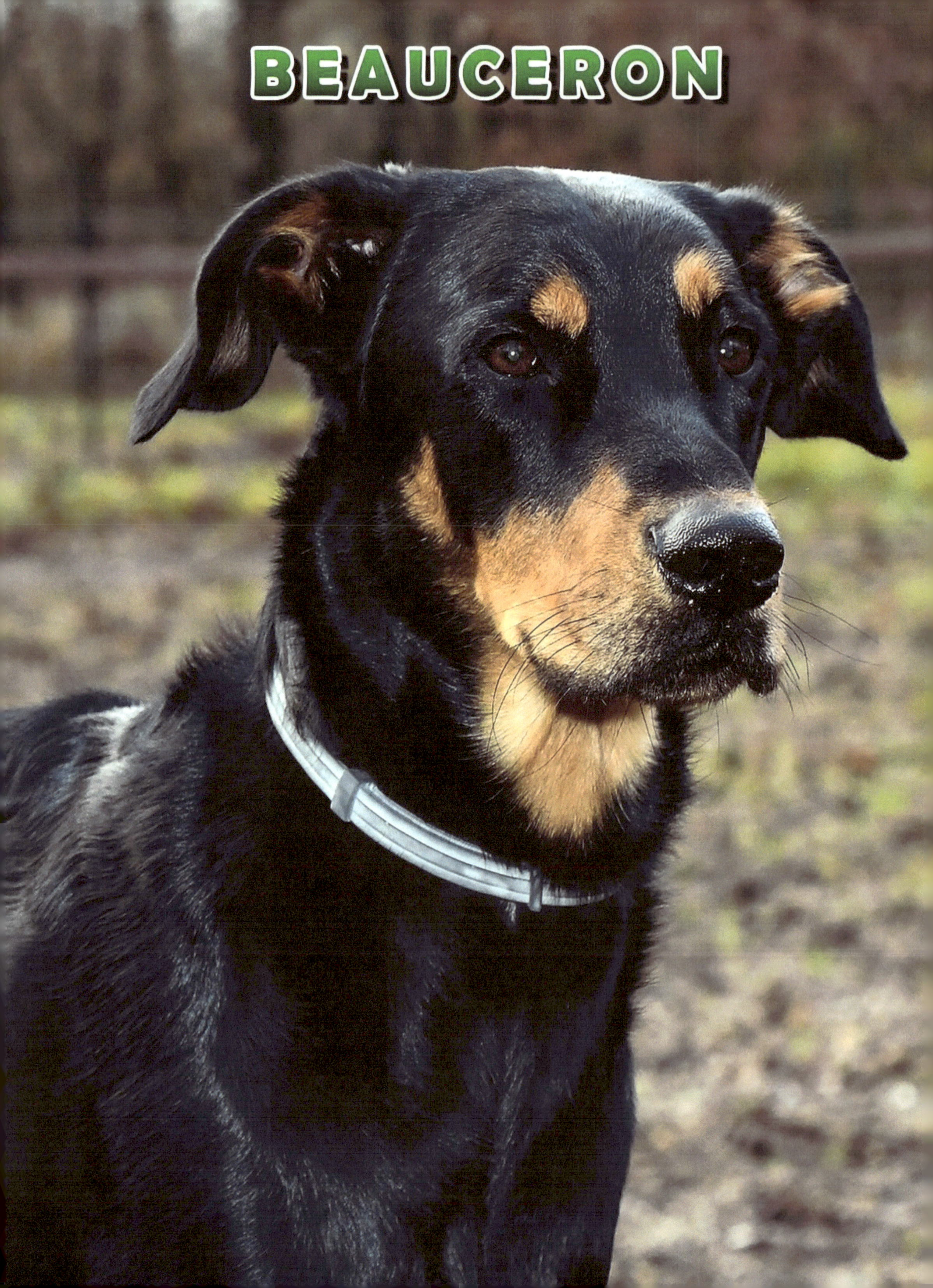

BLOODHOUND

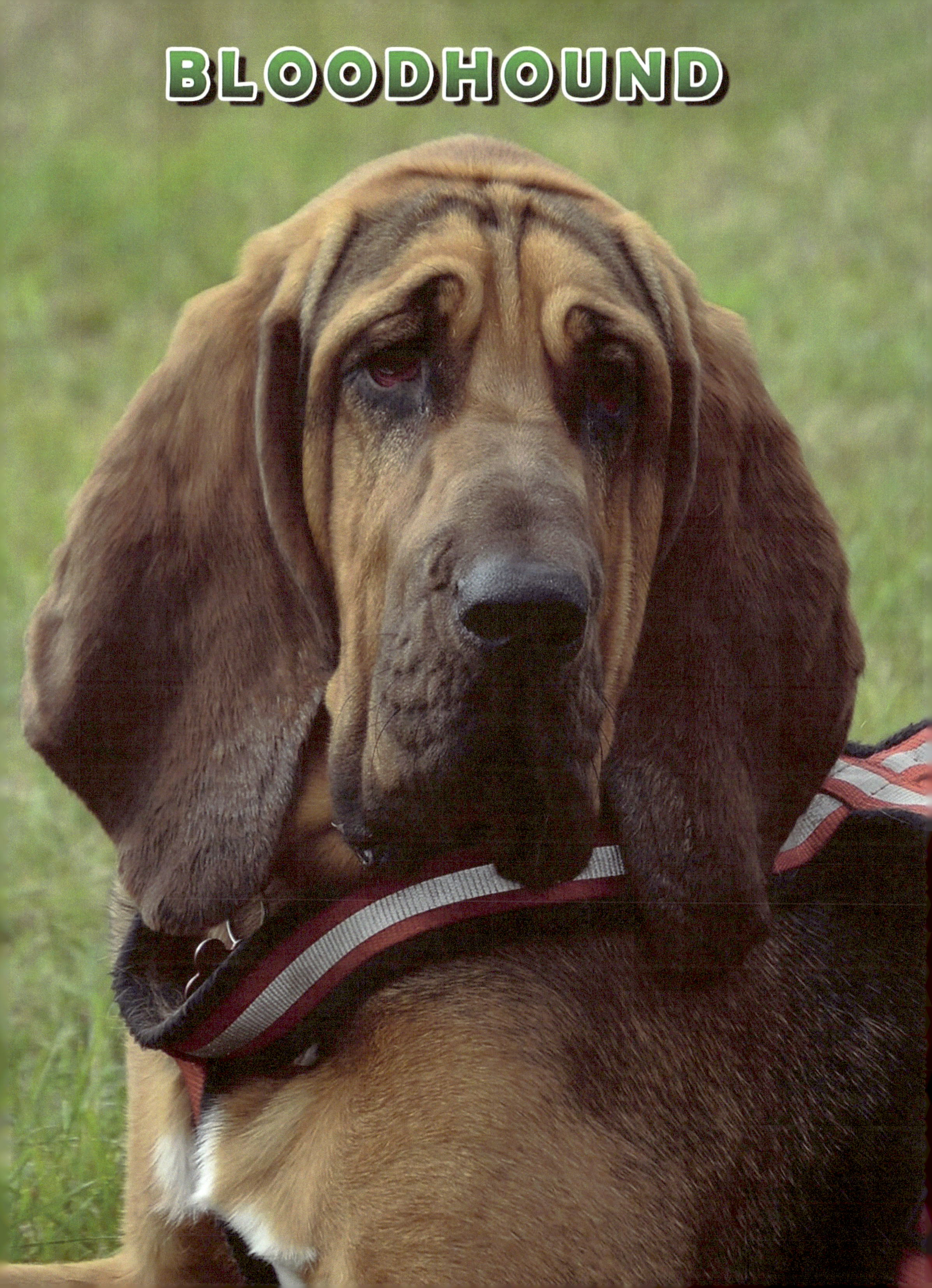

BORDER COLLIE

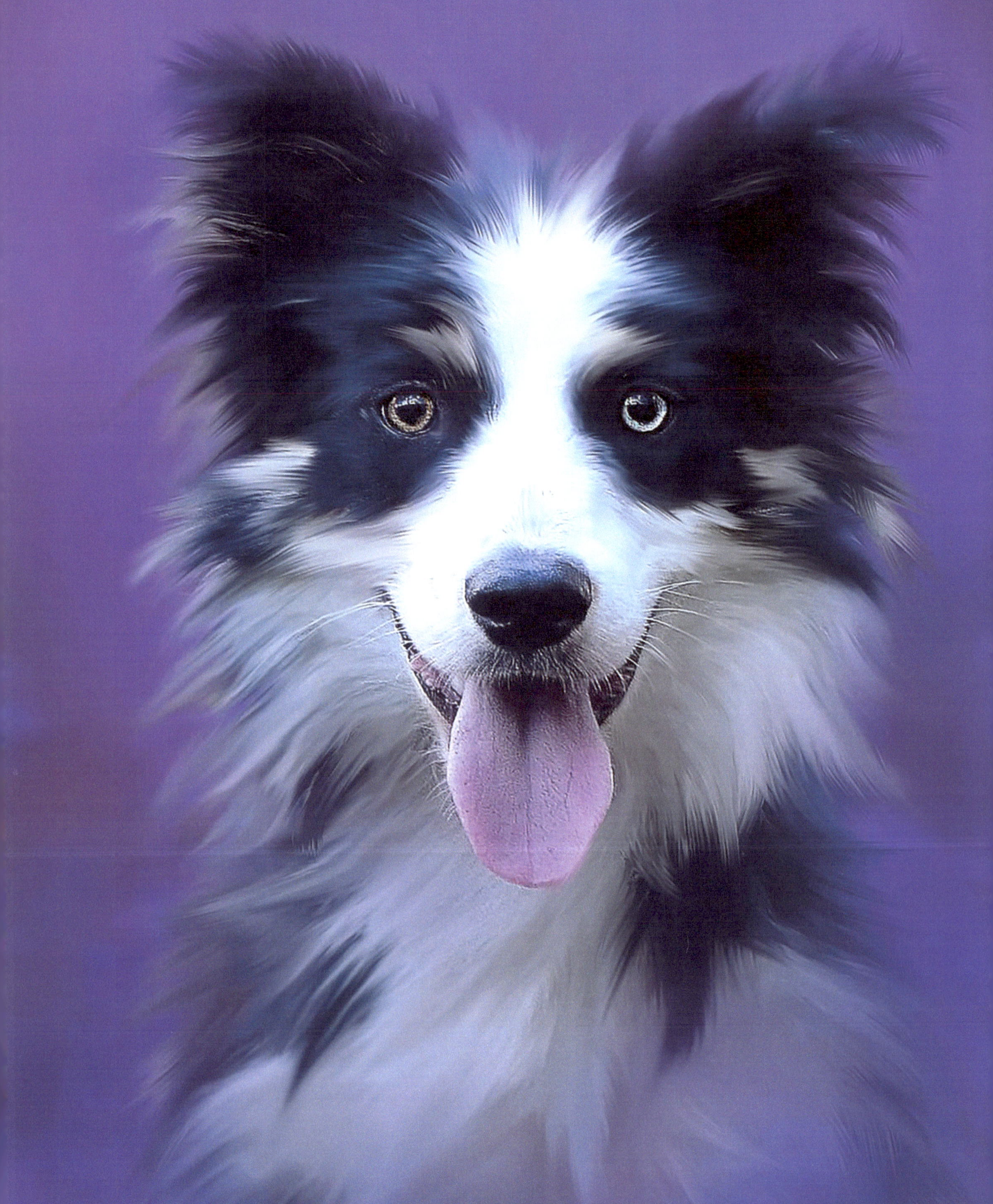

BOXER

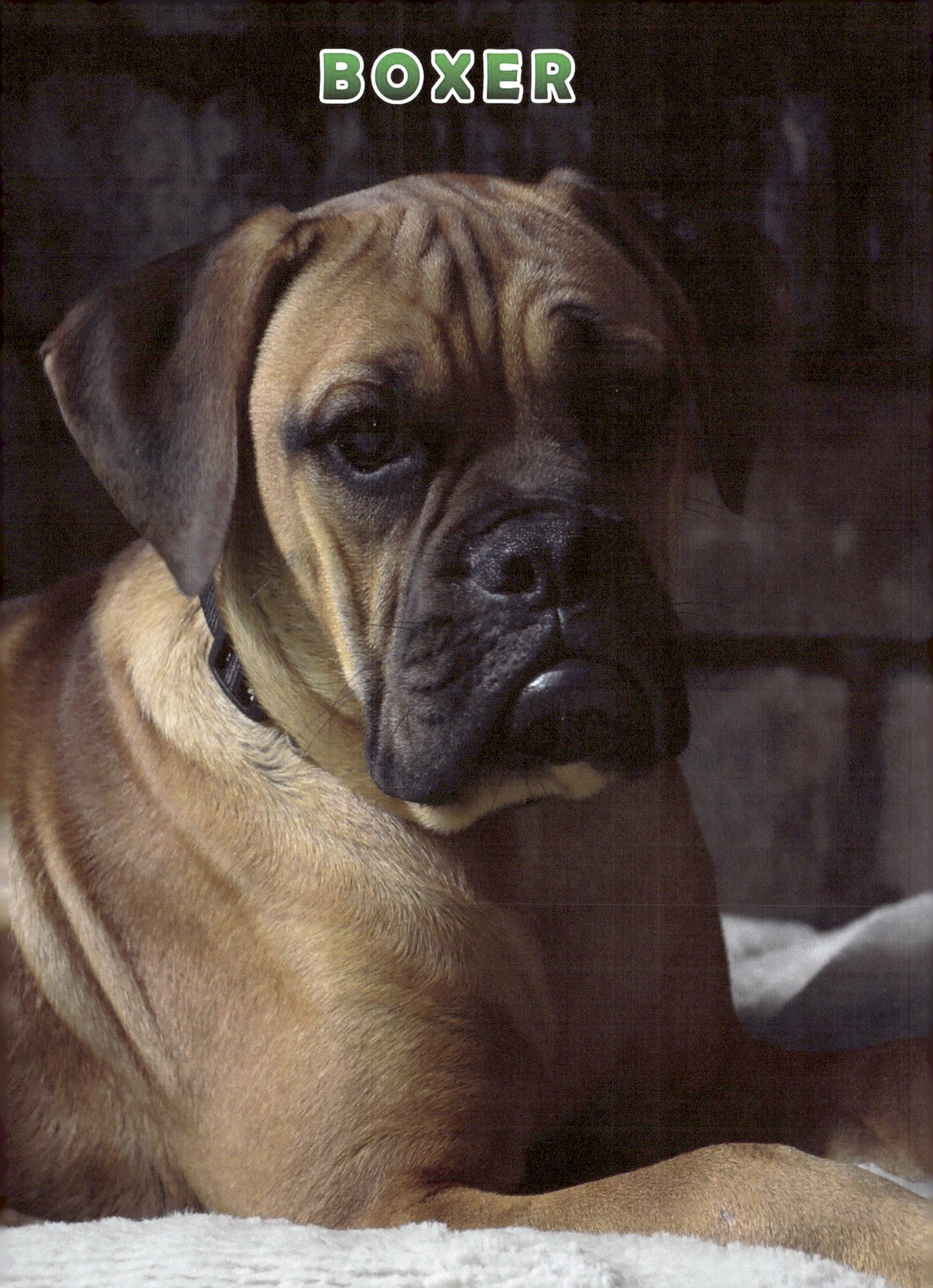

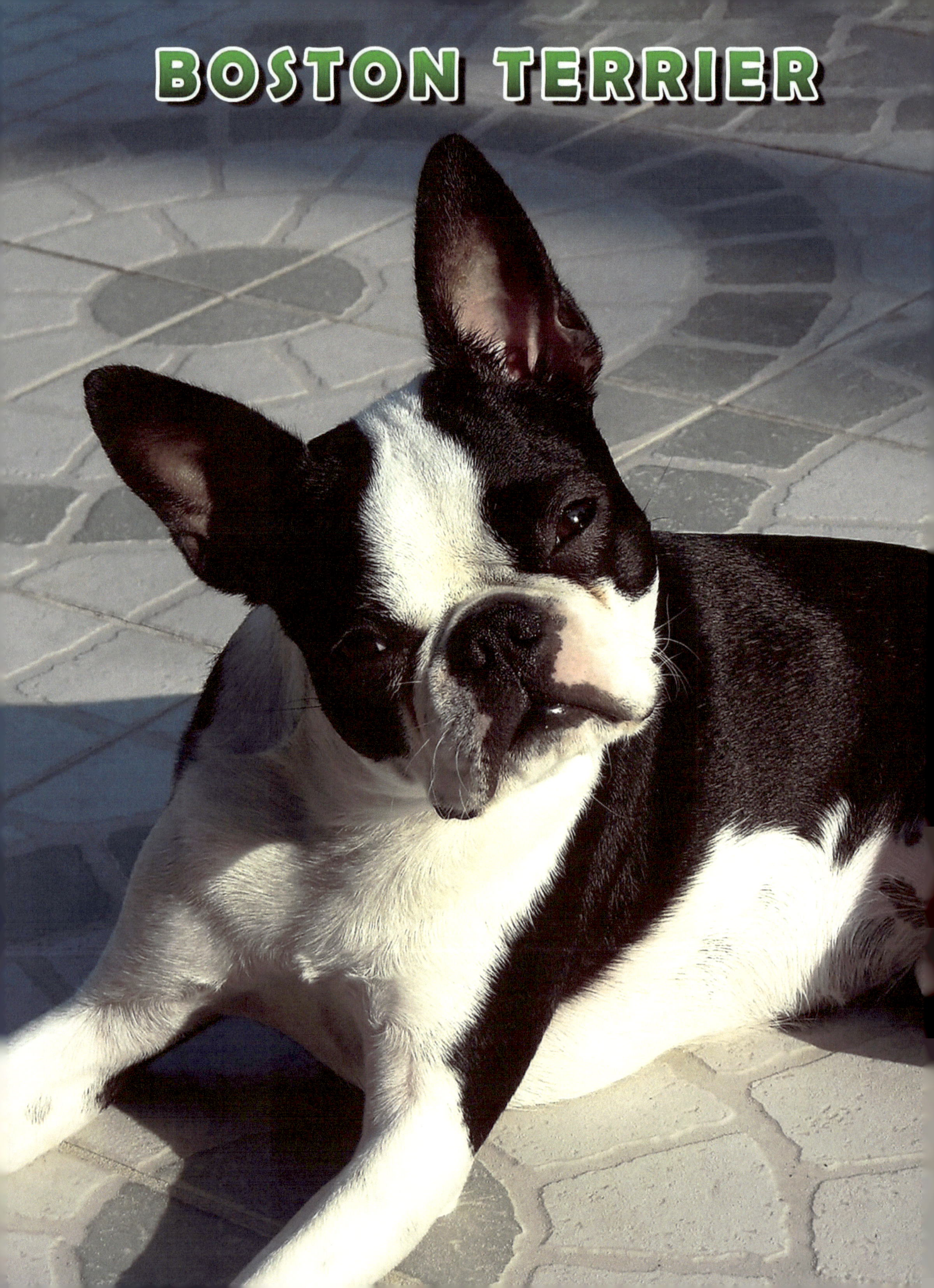

BOSTON TERRIER

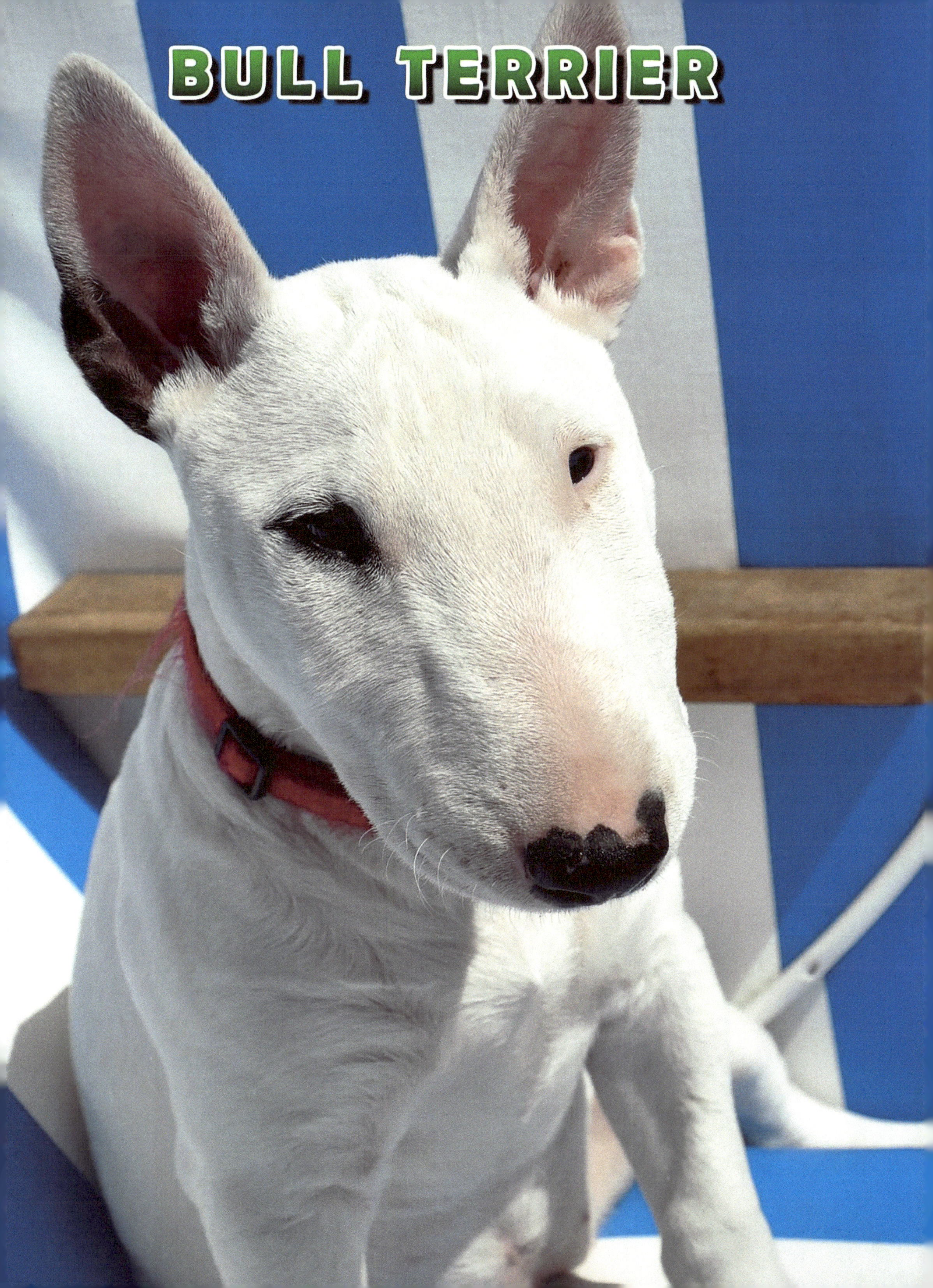

BULL TERRIER

CAVALIER KING CHARLES SPANIEL

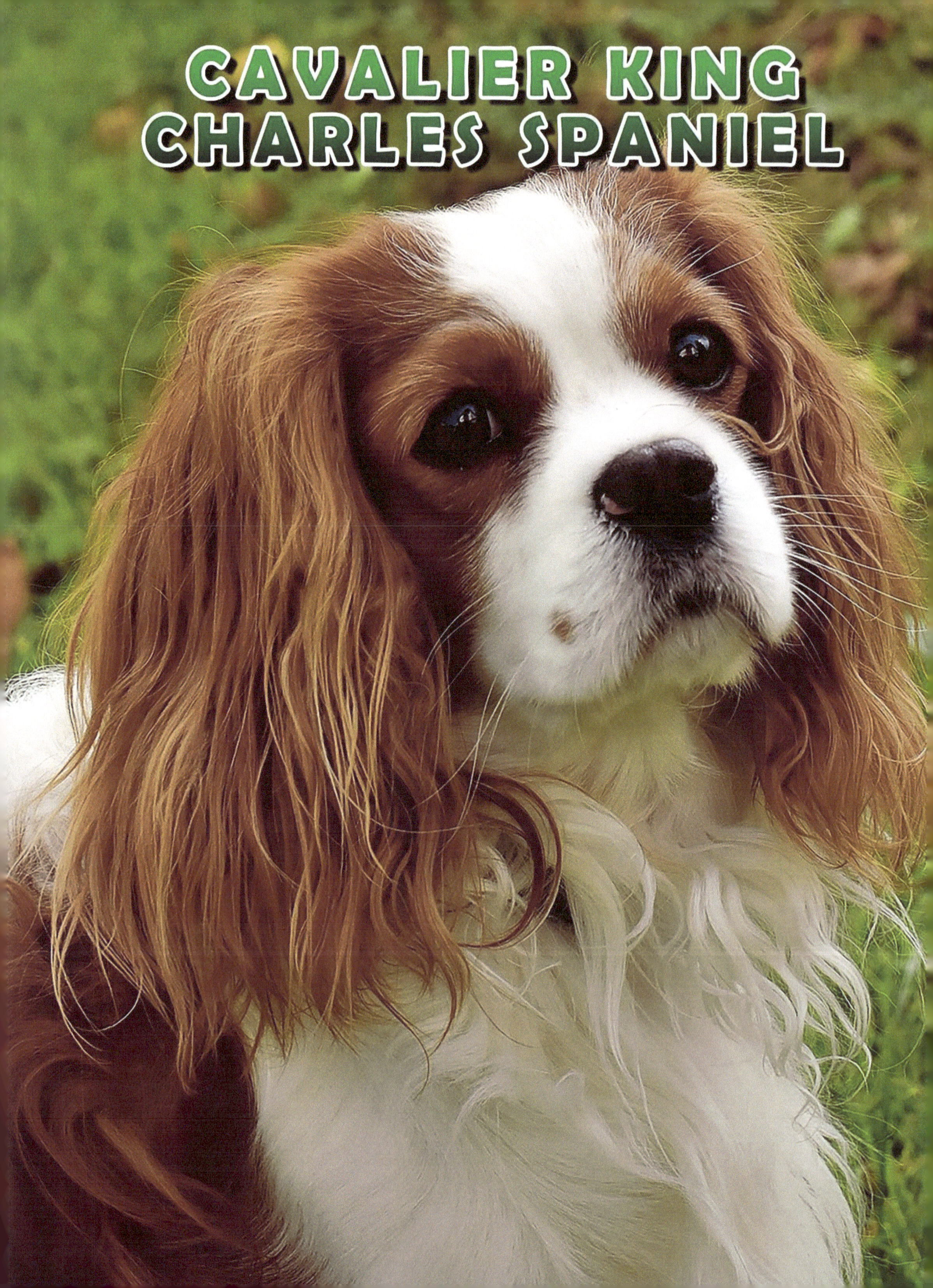

CHIHUAHUA

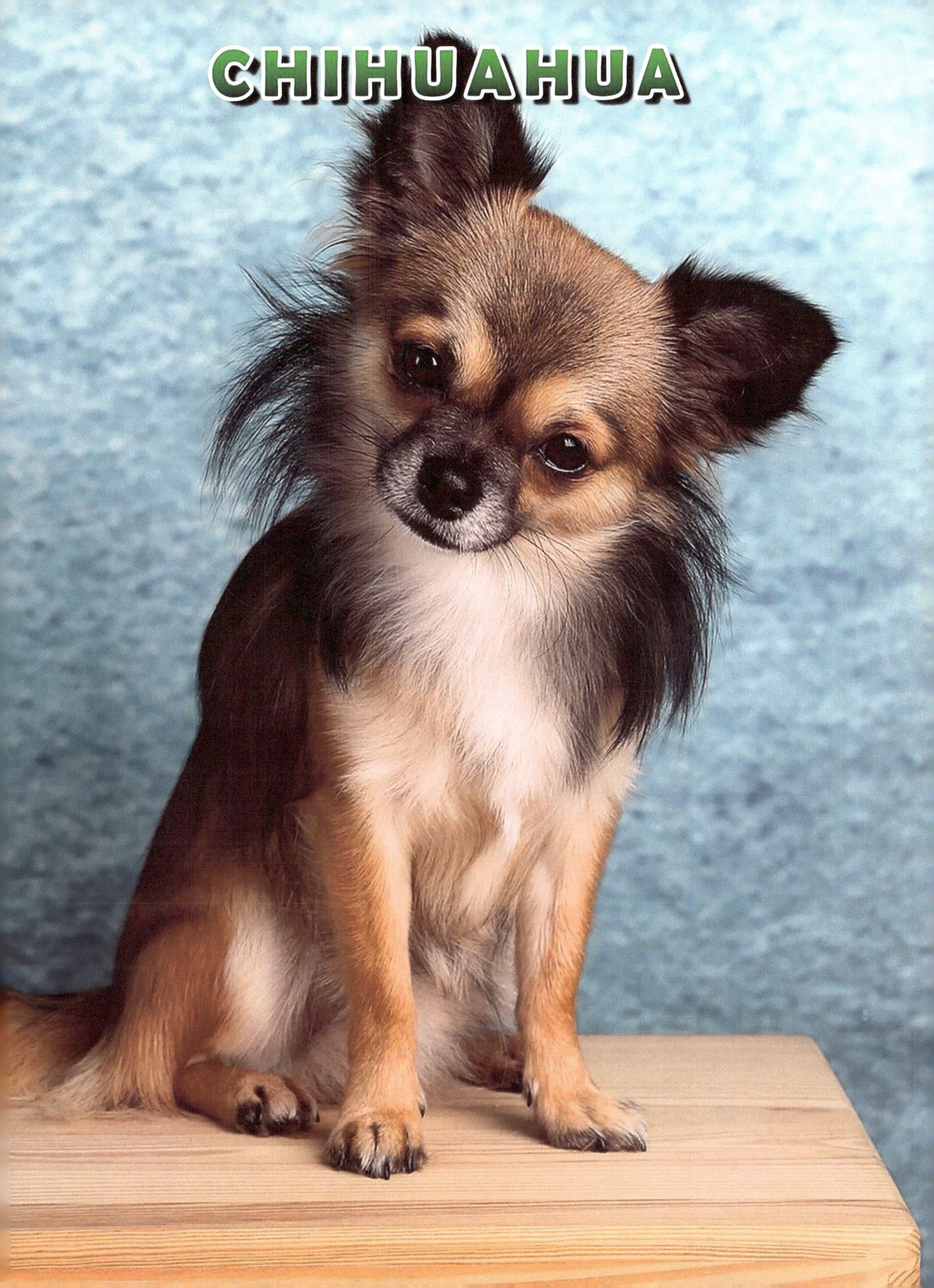

CHINESE CRESTED DOG

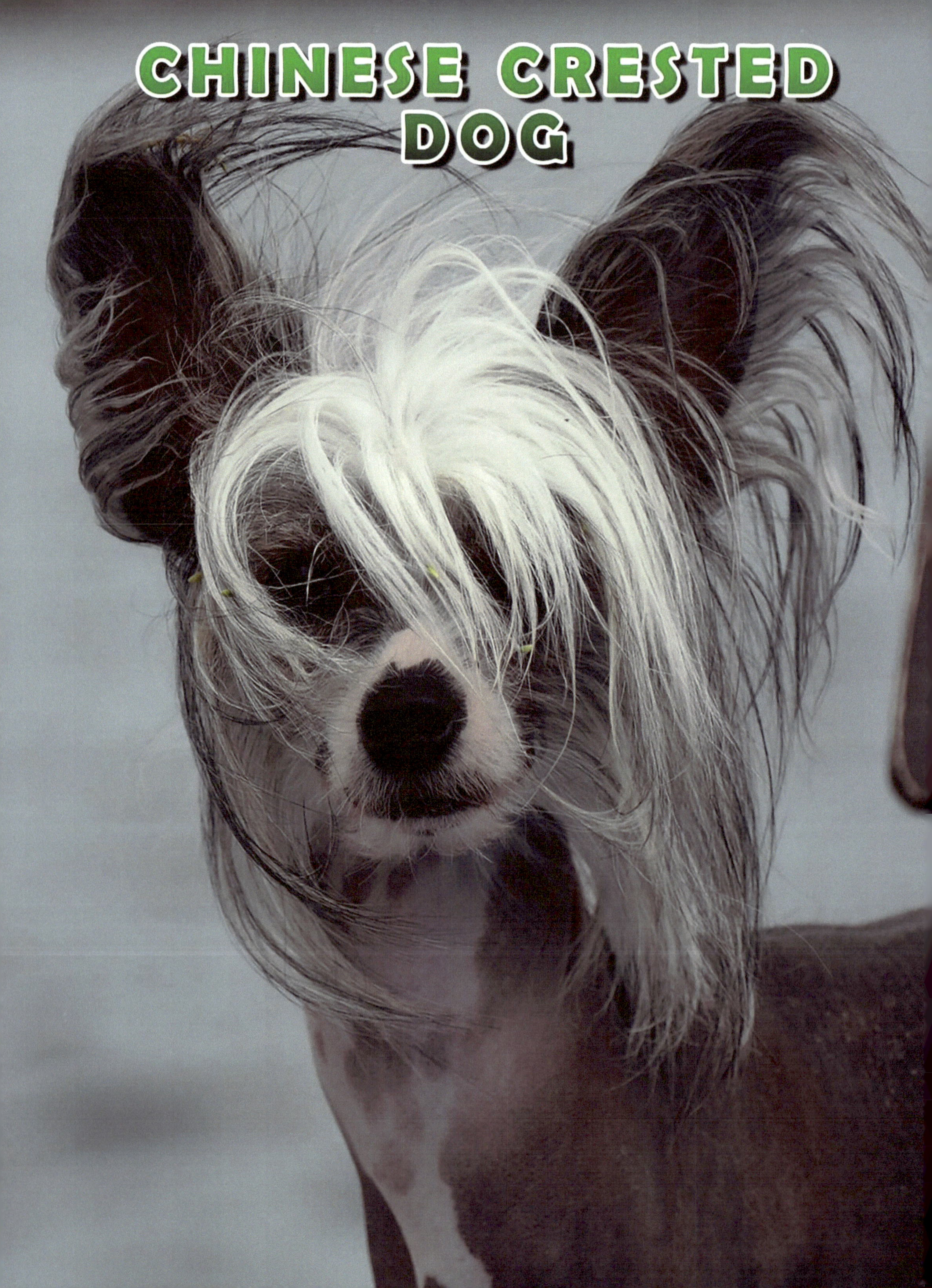

ENGLISH COCKER SPANIEL

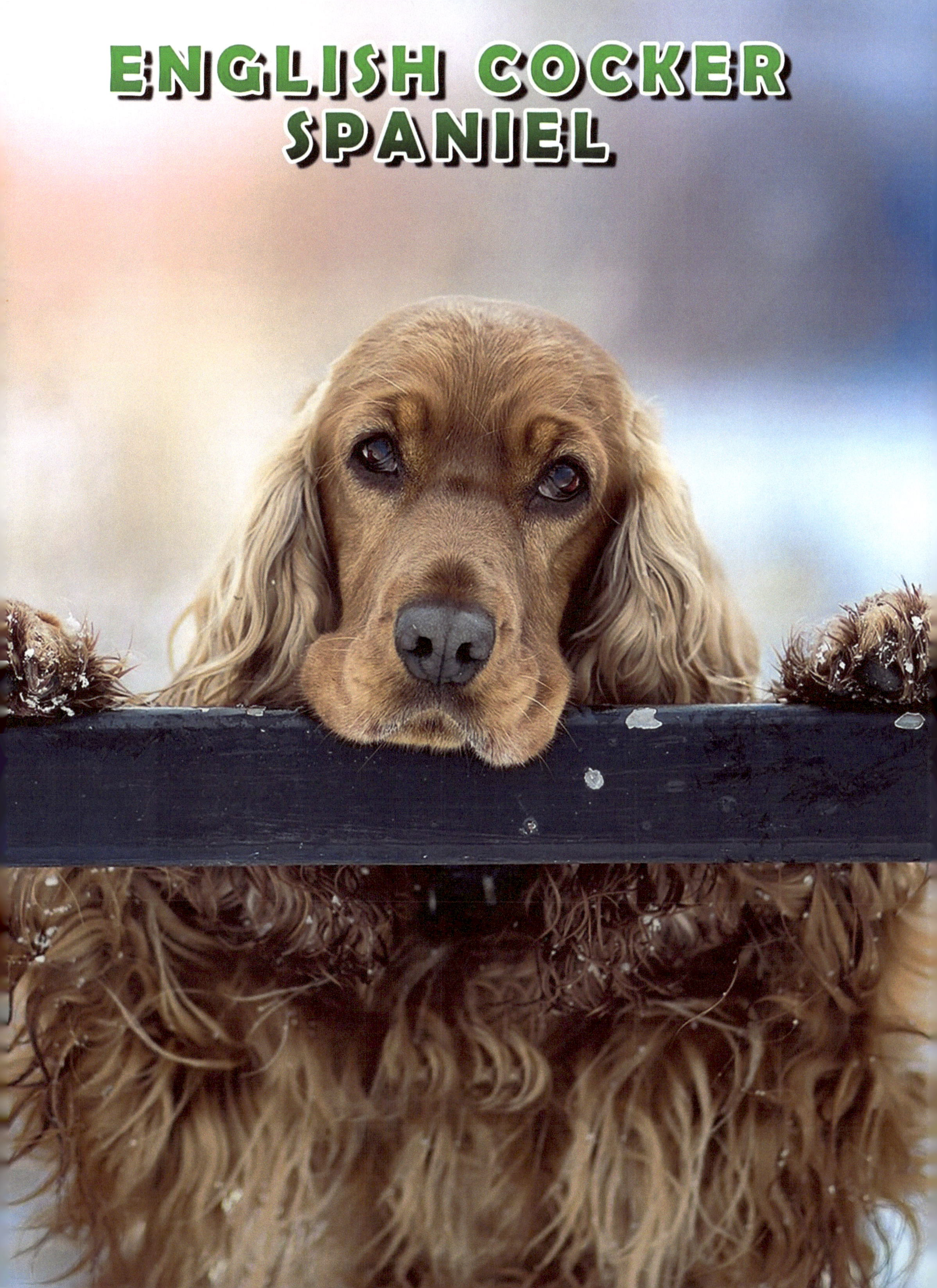

DACHSHUND PUPPY

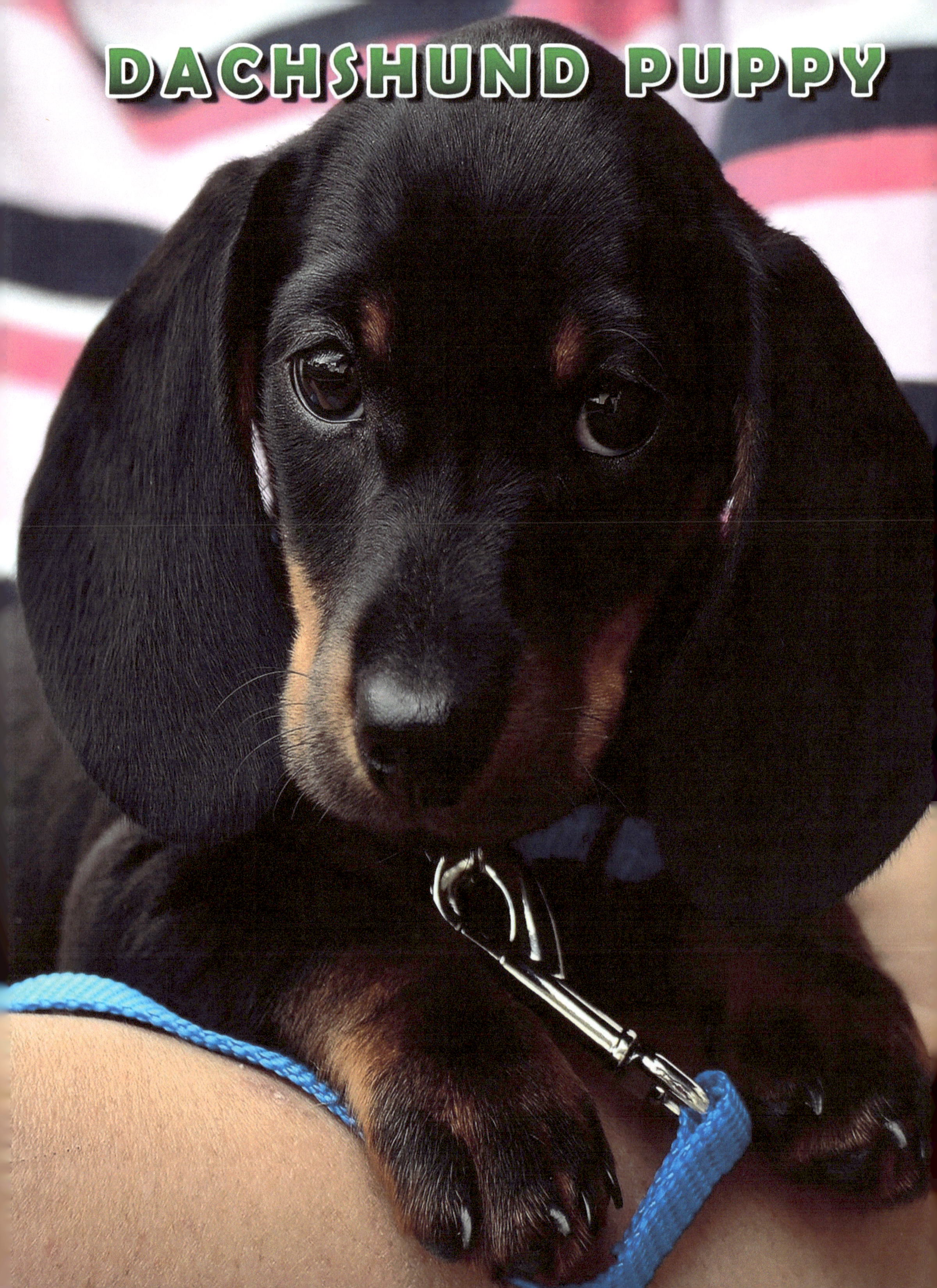

DALMATIAN

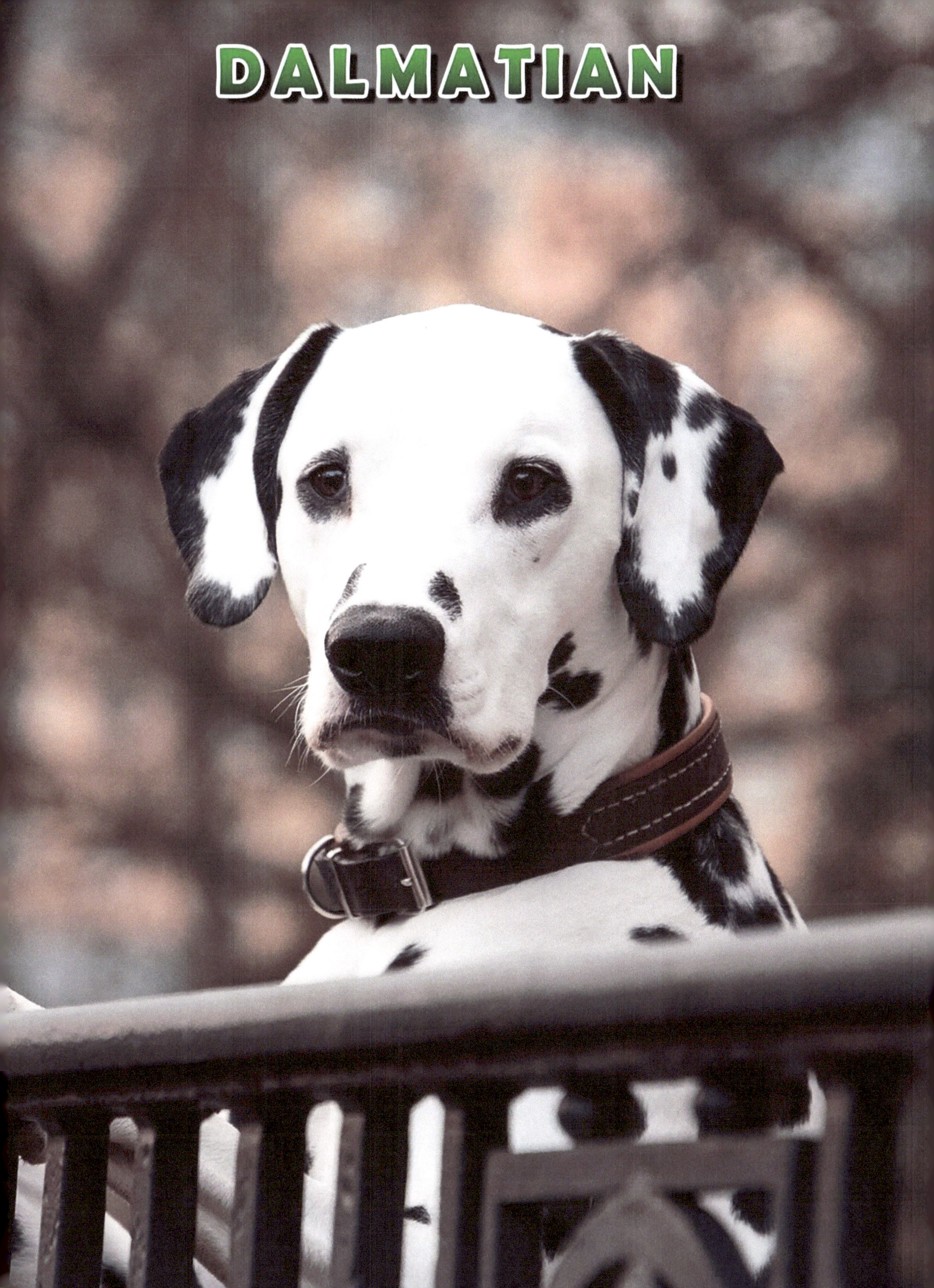

DOBERMAN PINSCHER

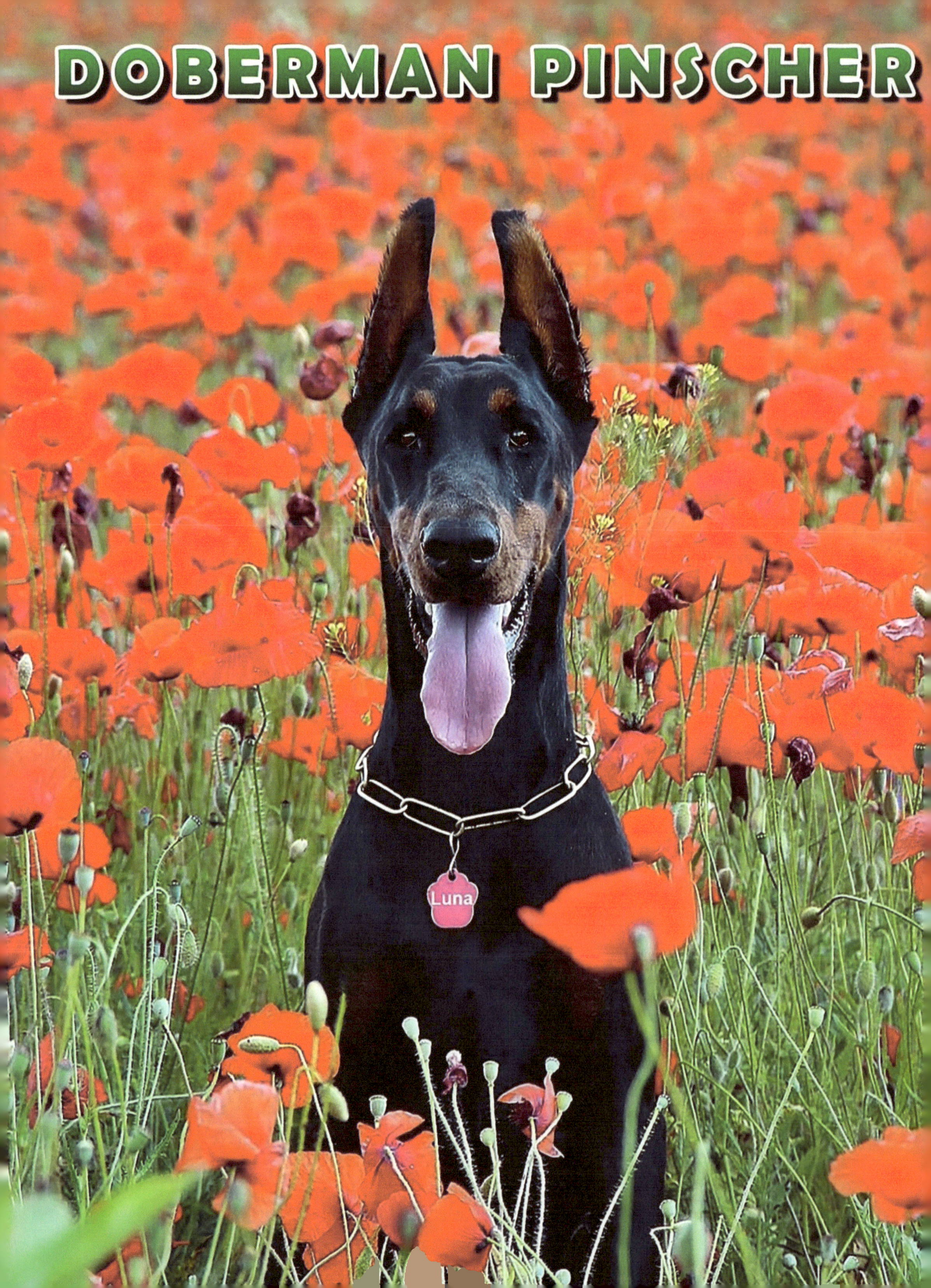

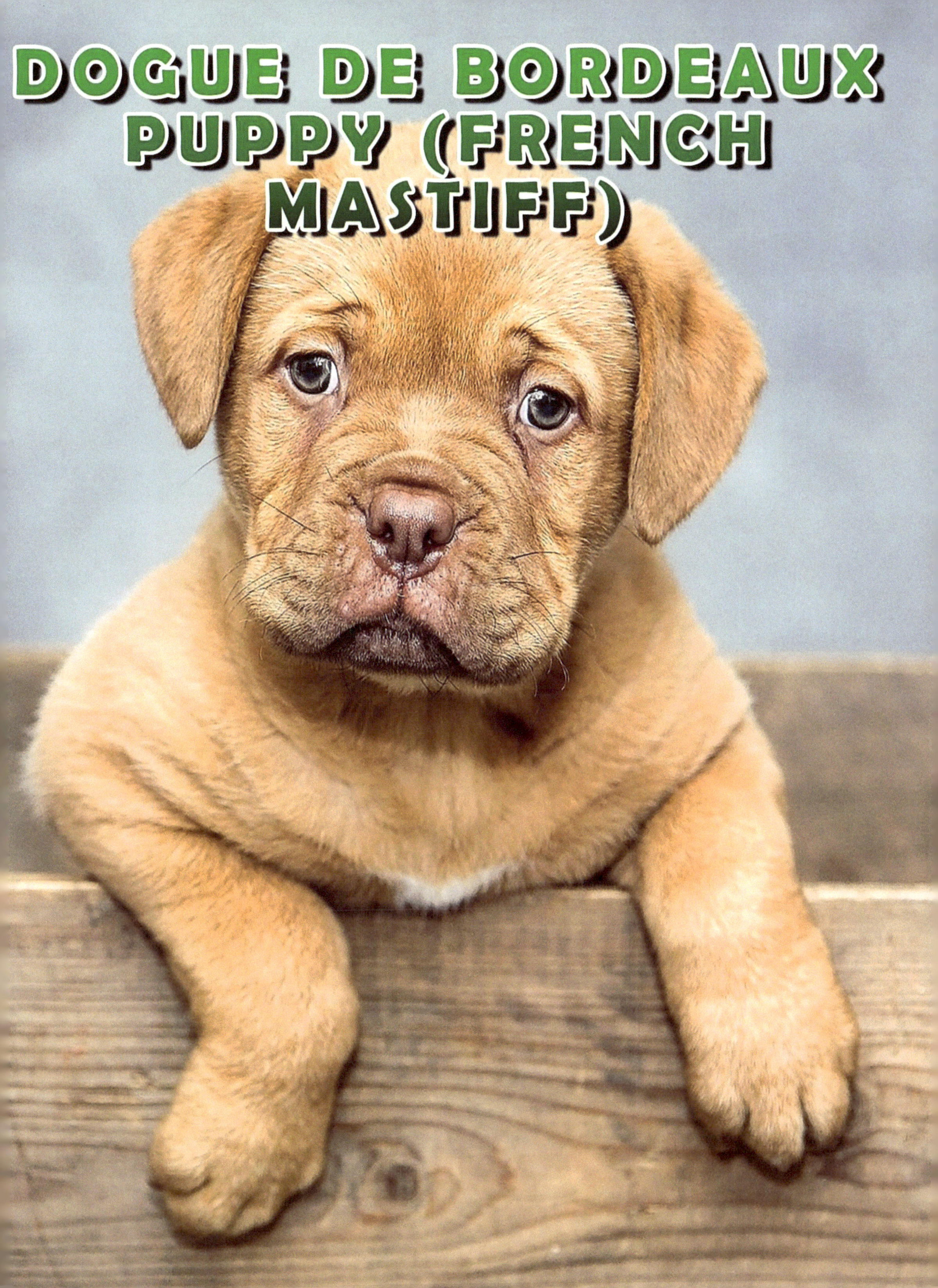
DOGUE DE BORDEAUX PUPPY (FRENCH MASTIFF)

ENGLISH BULLDOG

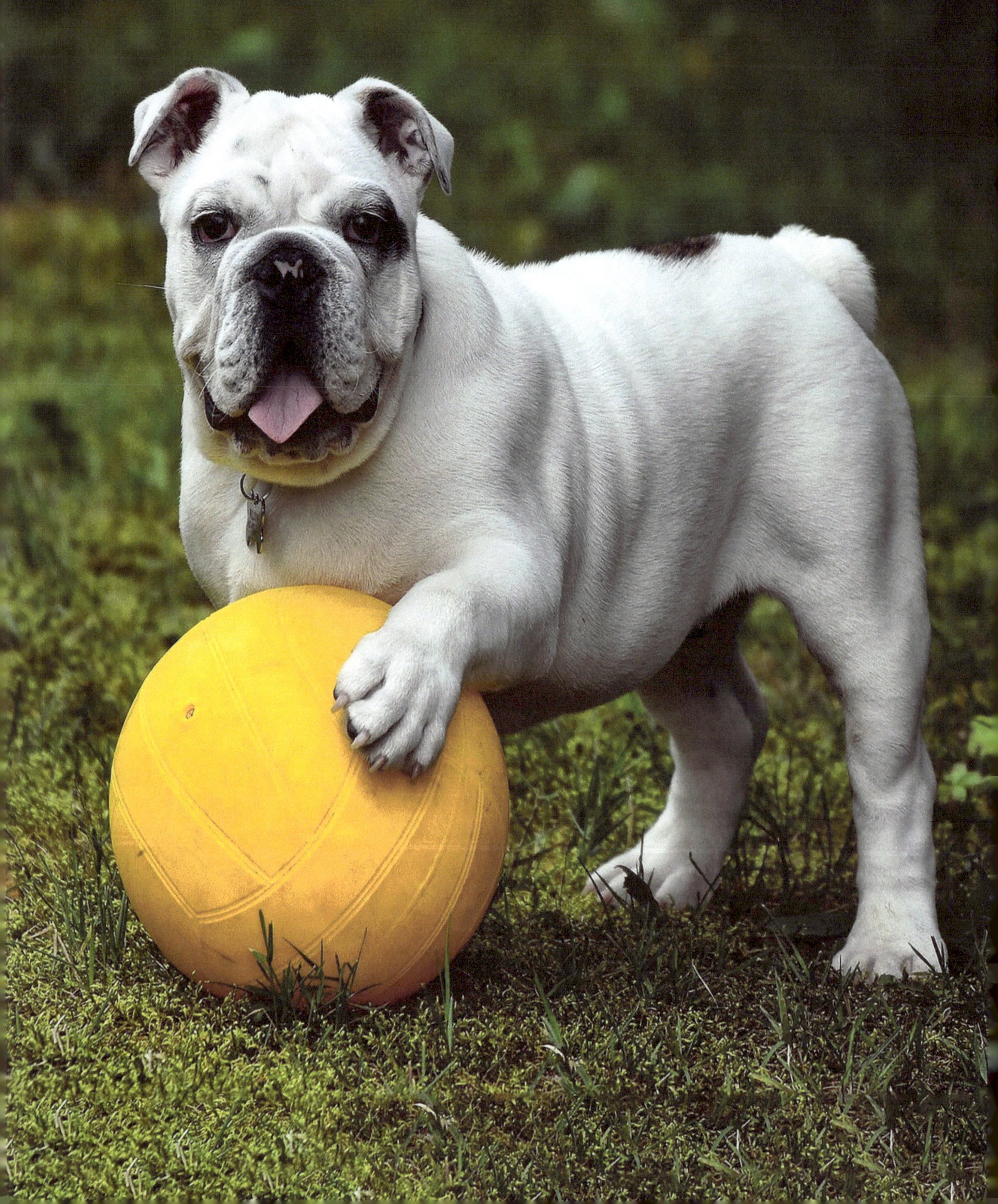

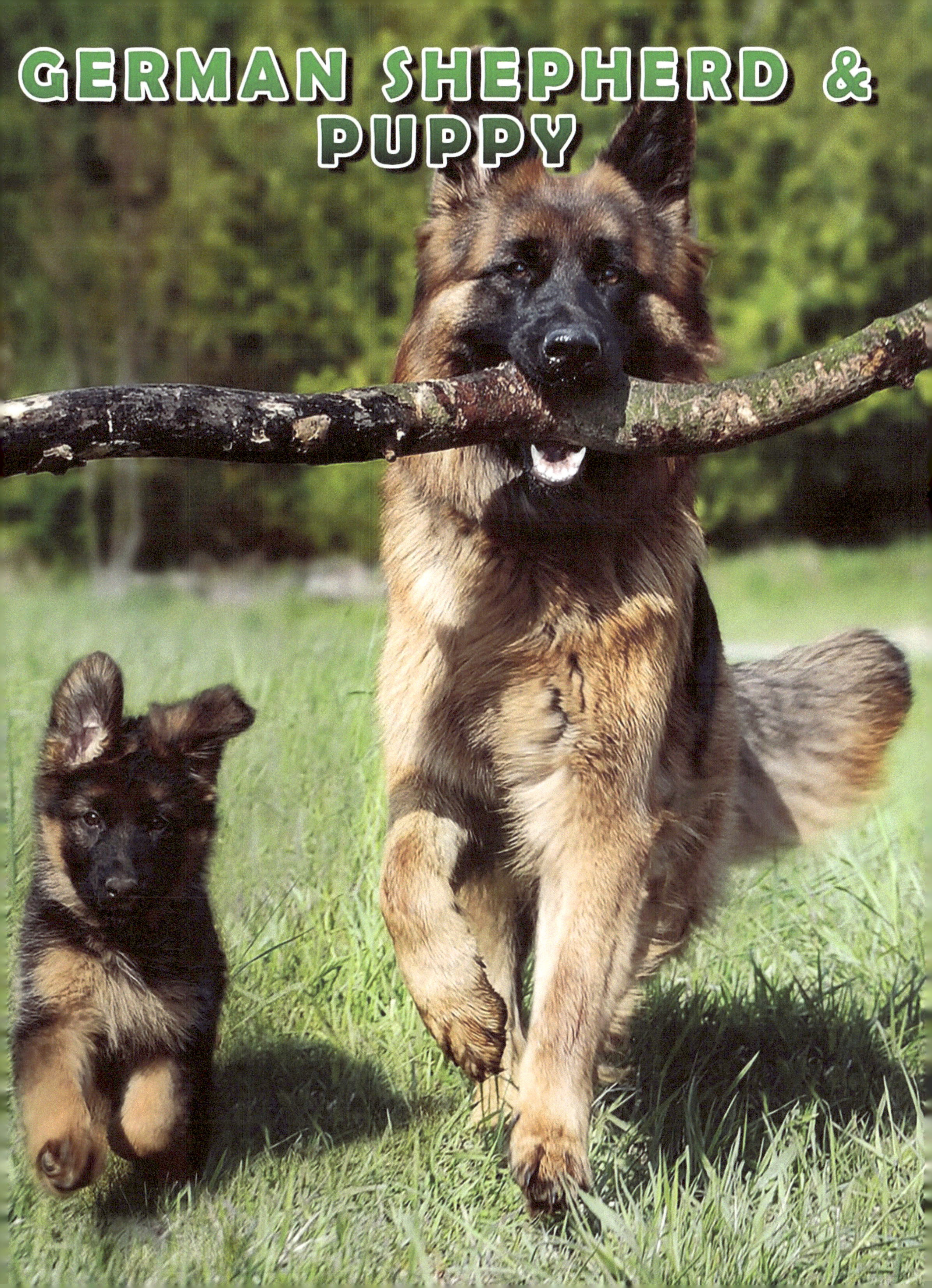

GERMAN SHEPHERD &
PUPPY

GOLDEN RETRIEVER

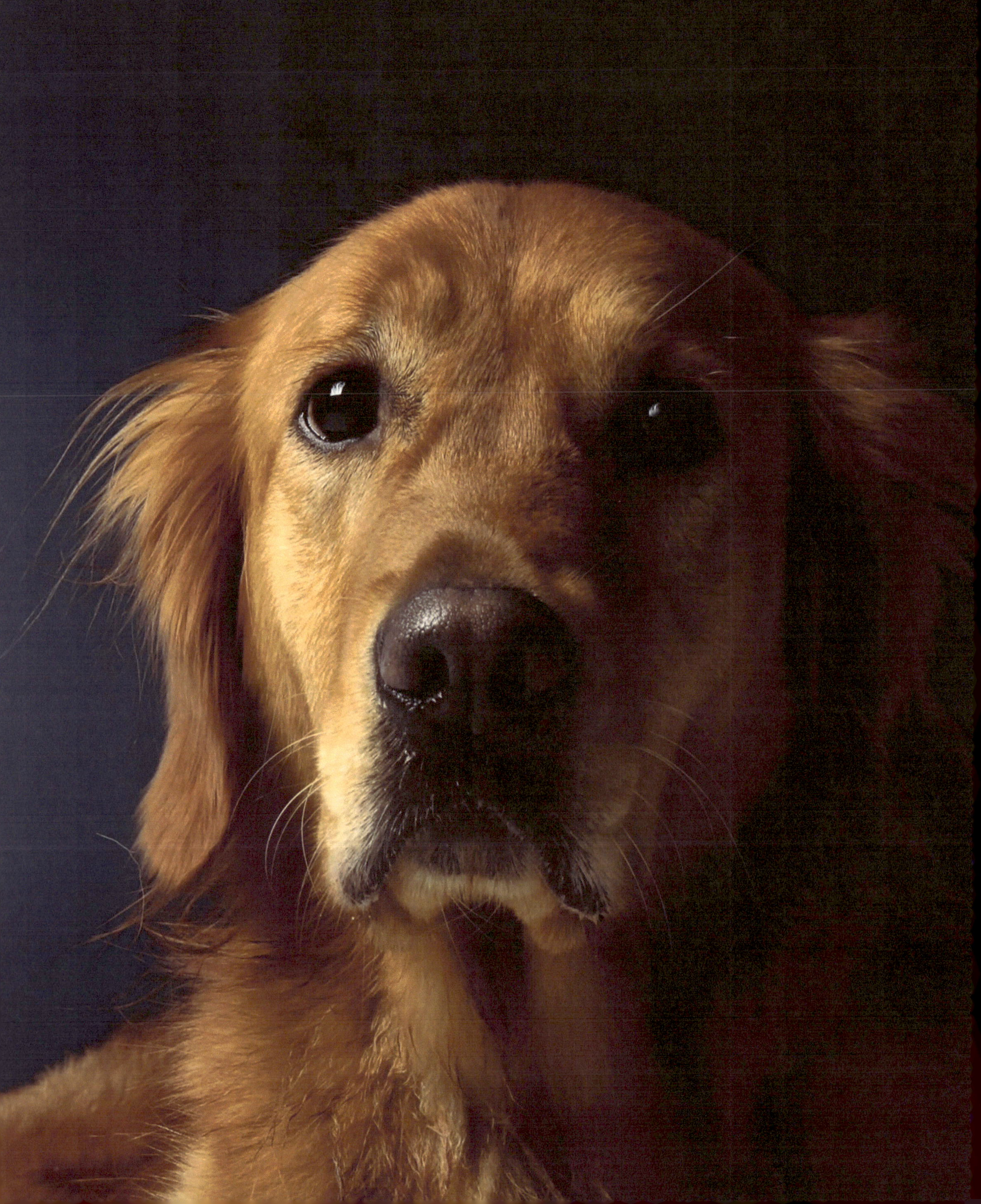

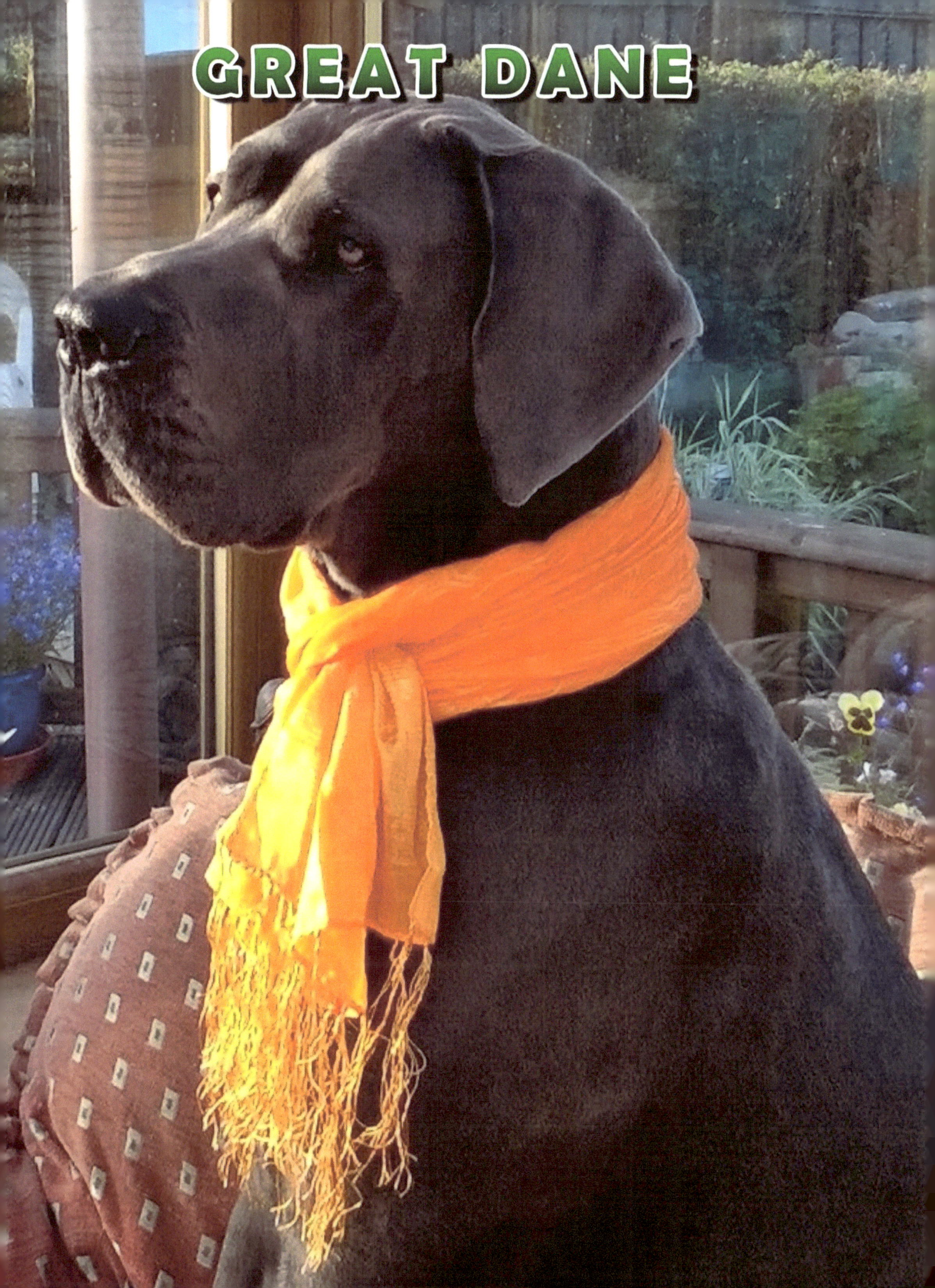
GREAT DANE

HAVANESE DOG

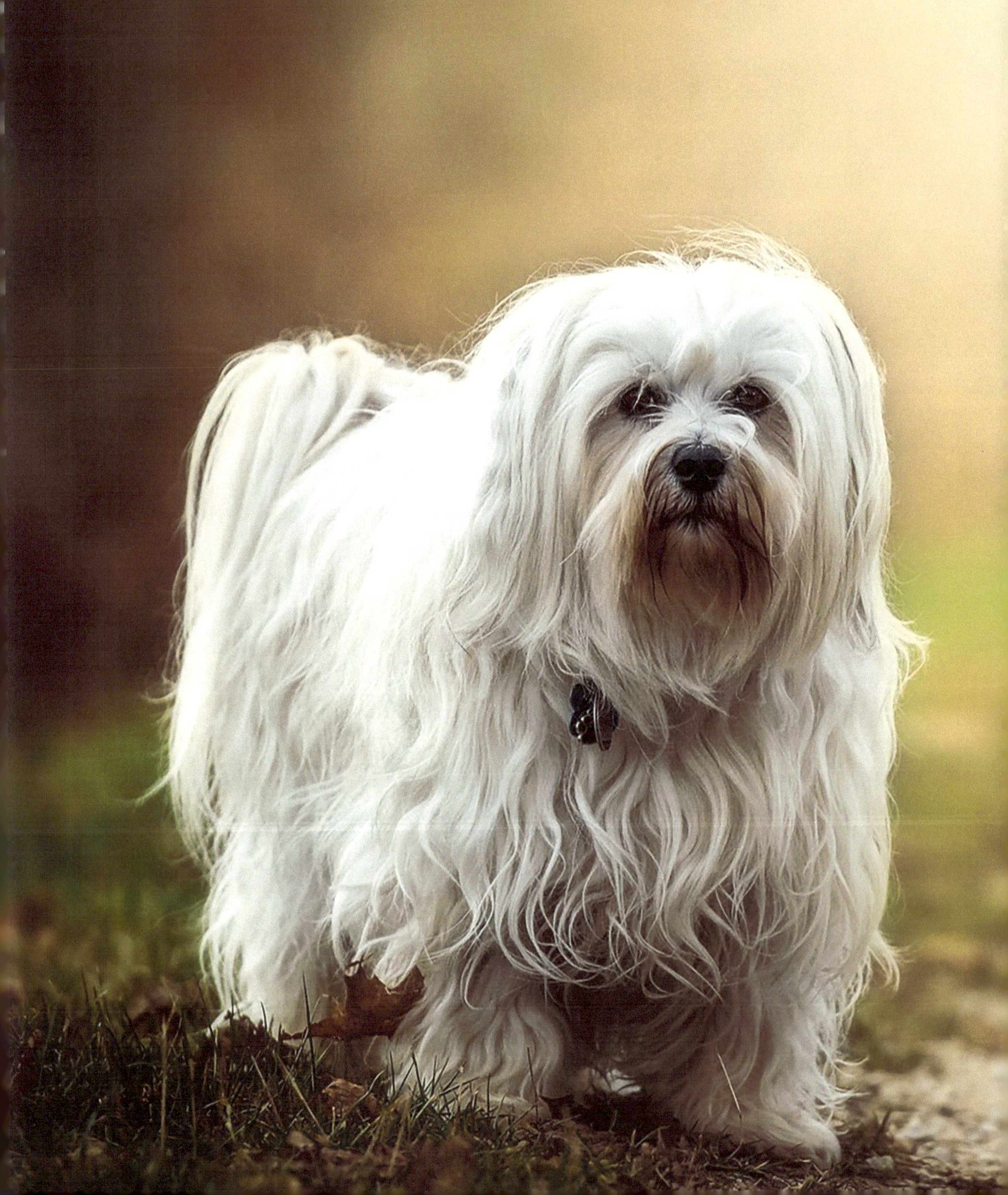

IRISH SETTER

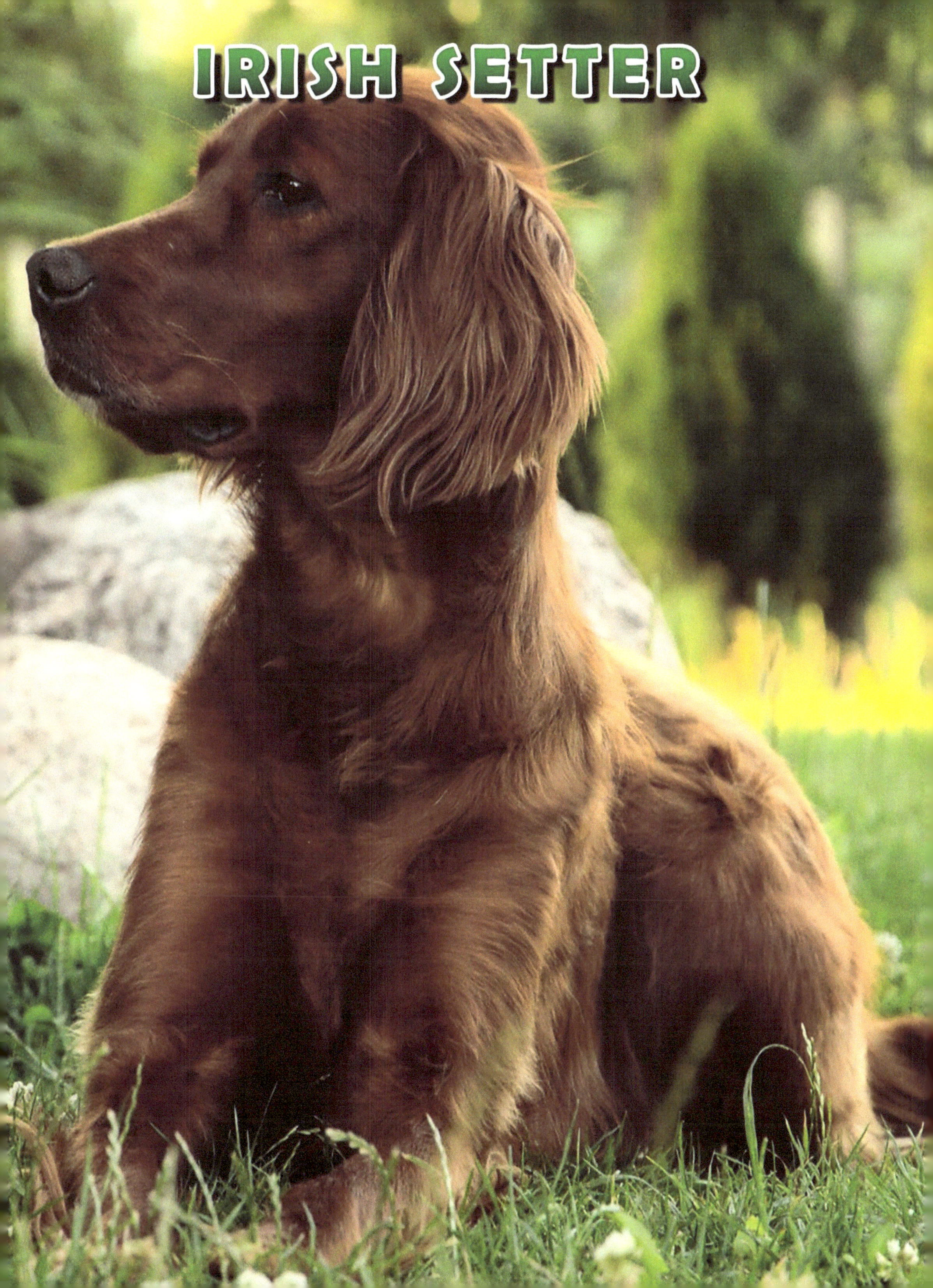

JACK RUSSELL TERRIER

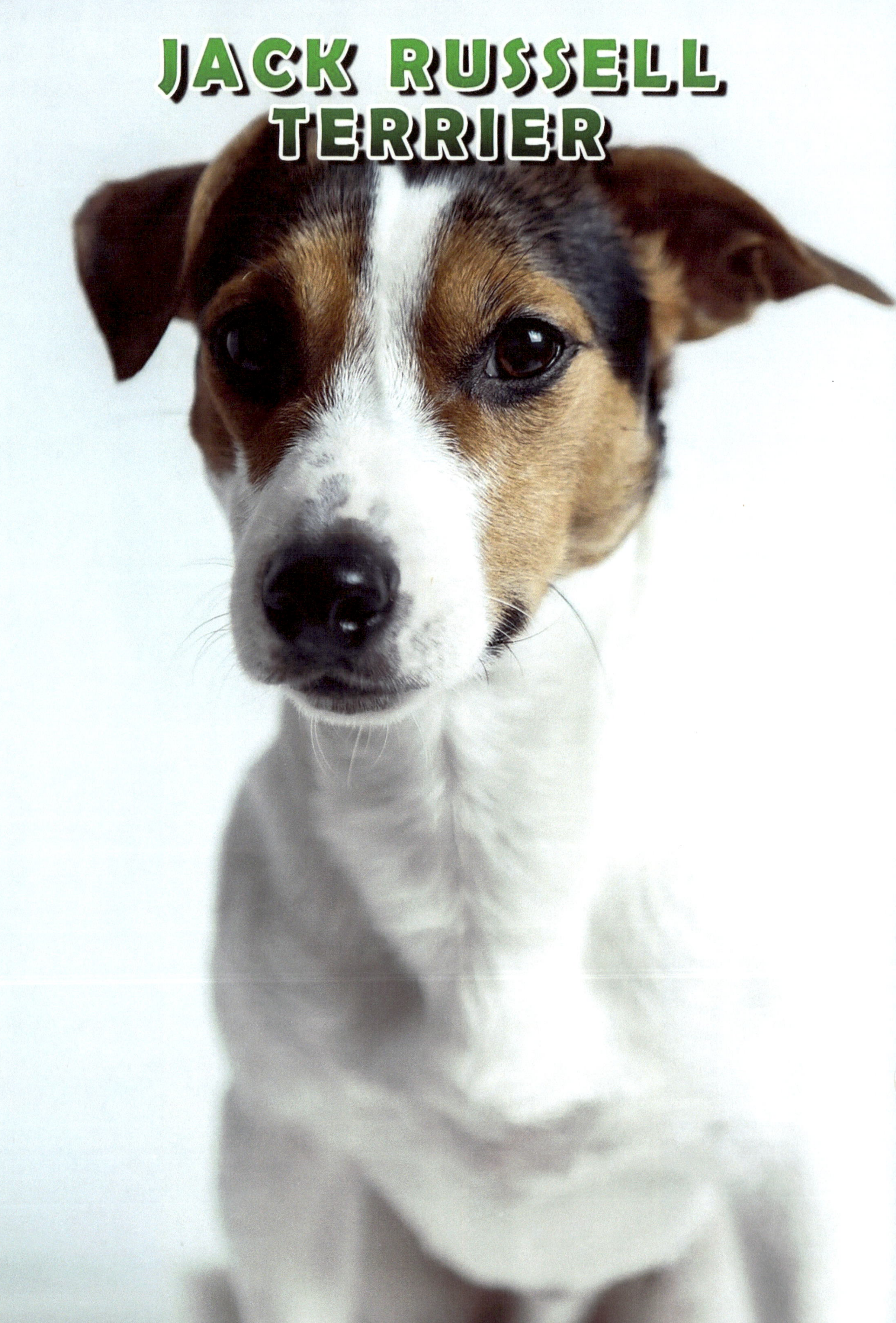

MALINOIS & BORDER COLLIE

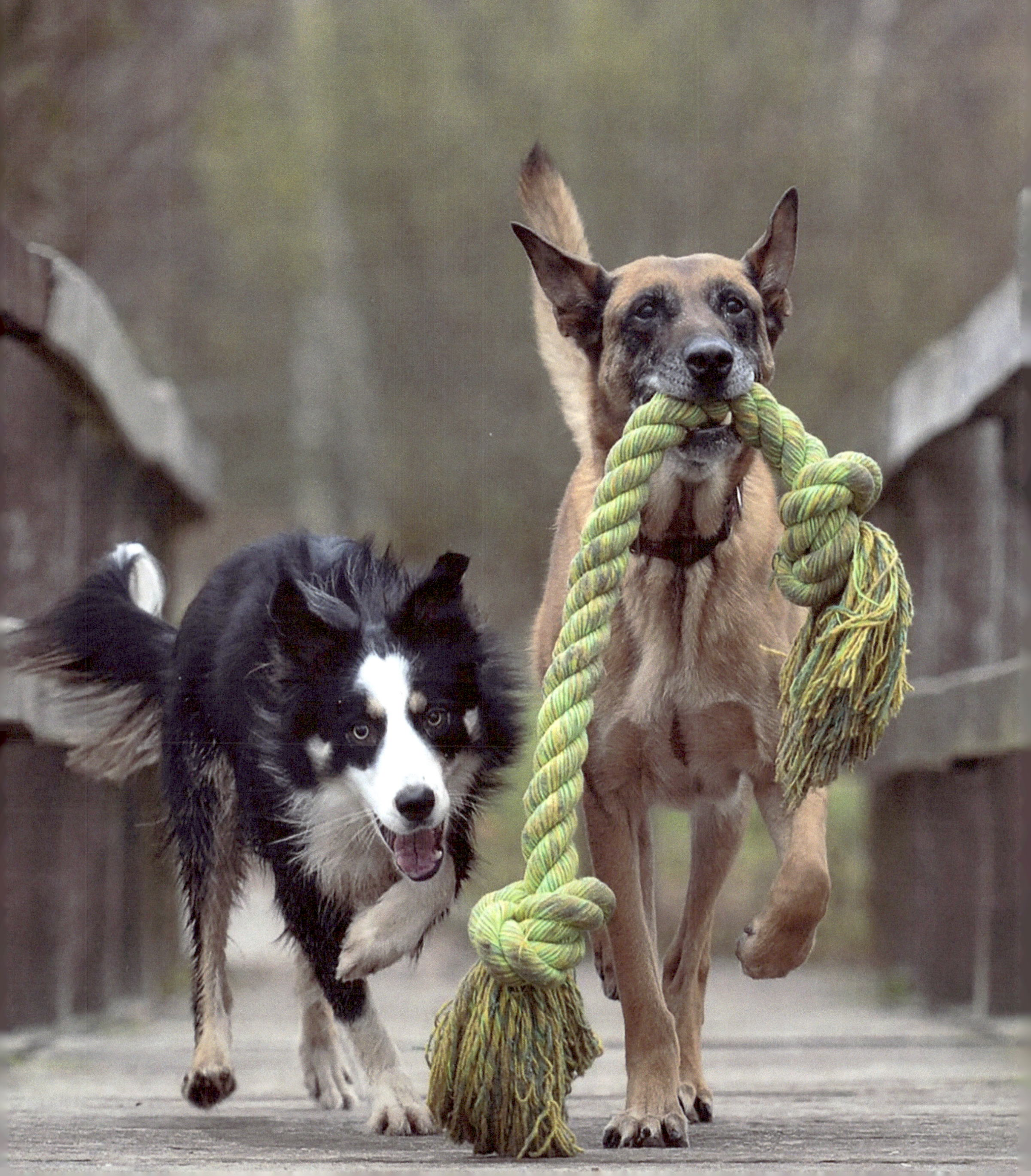

MALTESE POODLE PUPPY

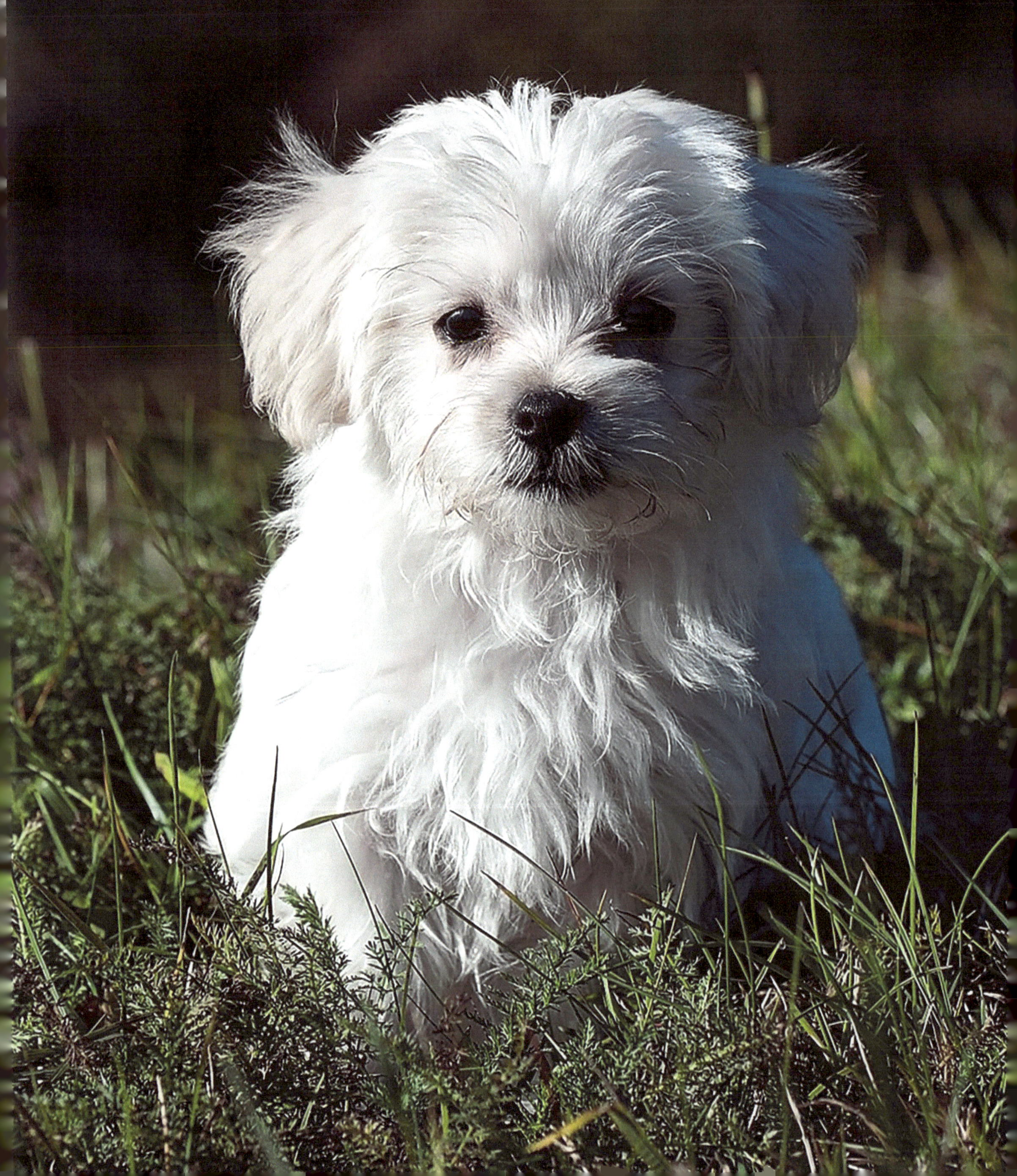

PEKINGESE

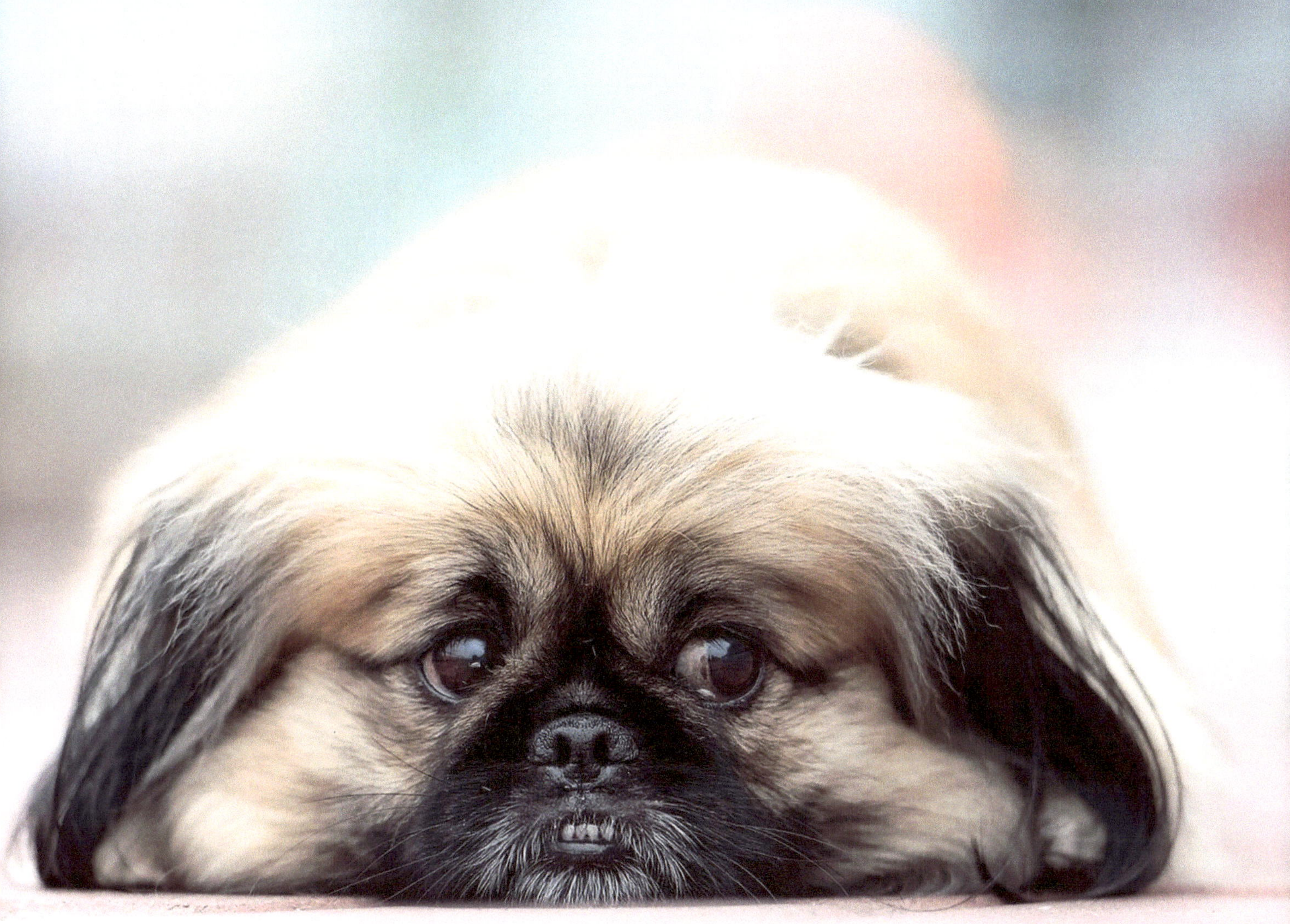

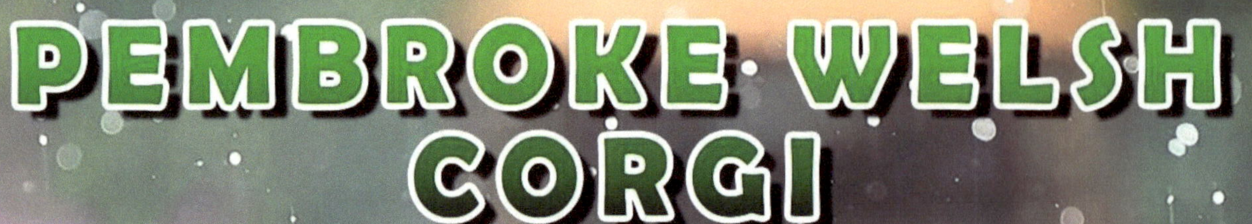
PEMBROKE WELSH
CORGI

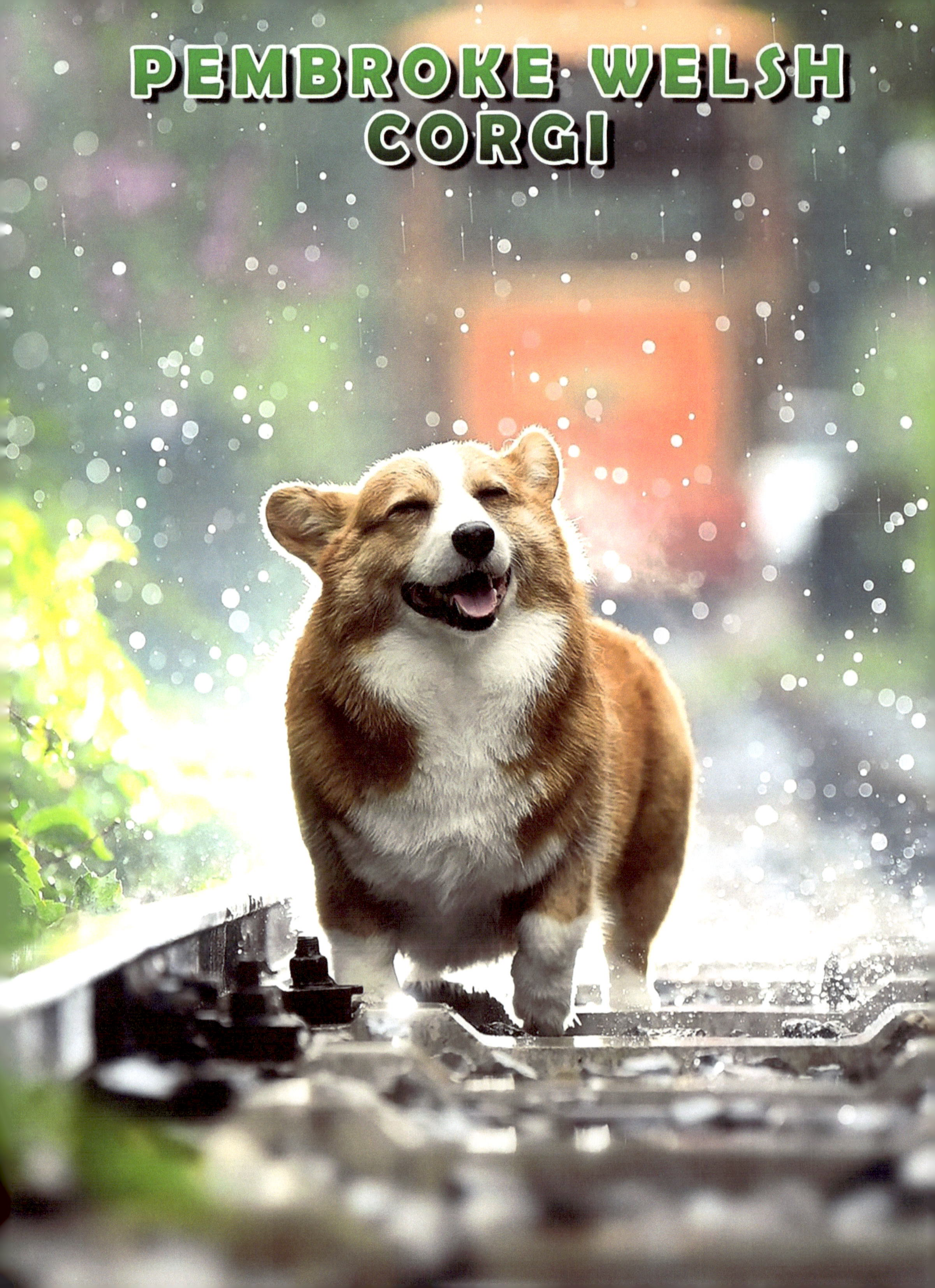

POMERANIAN

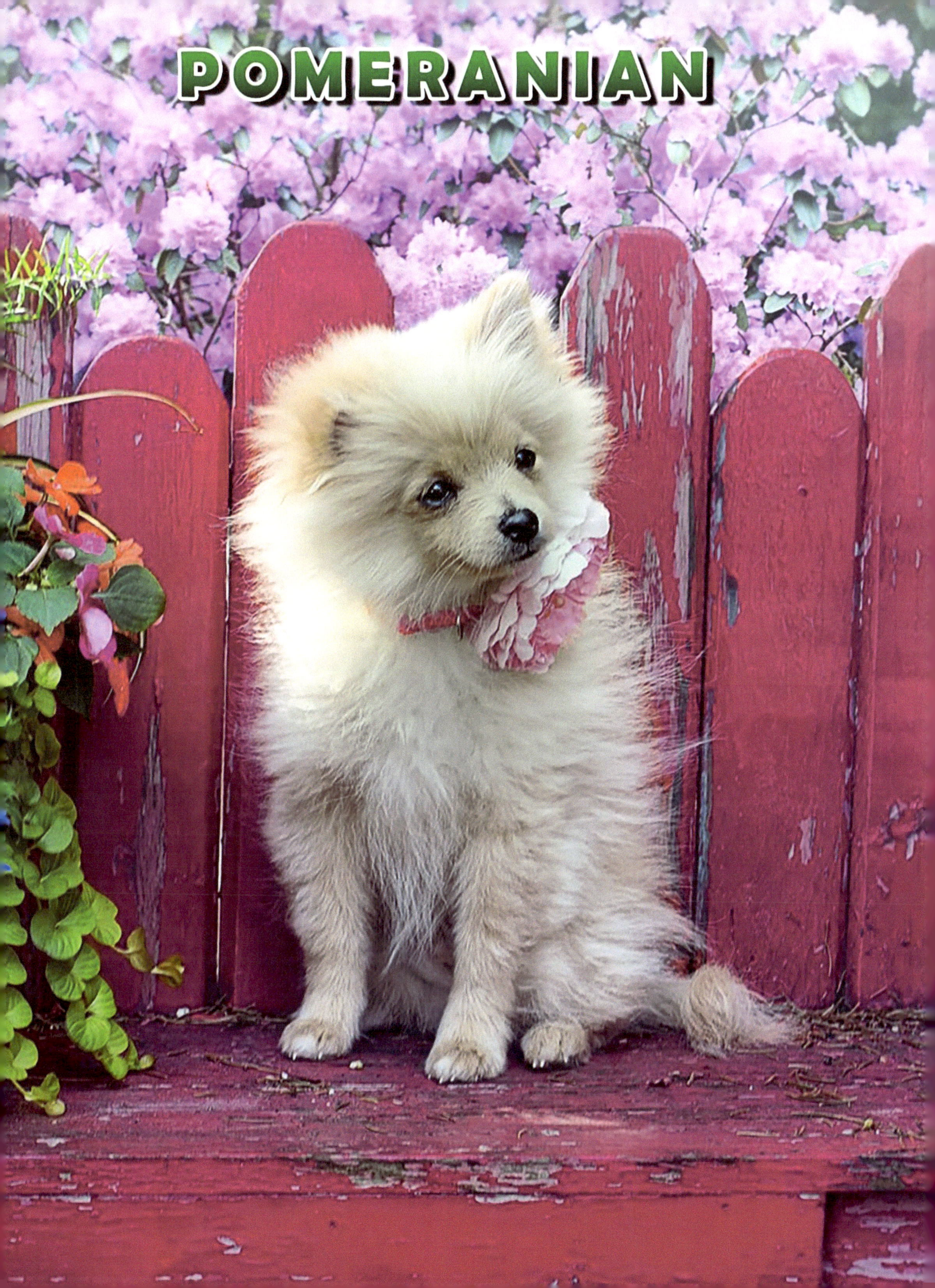

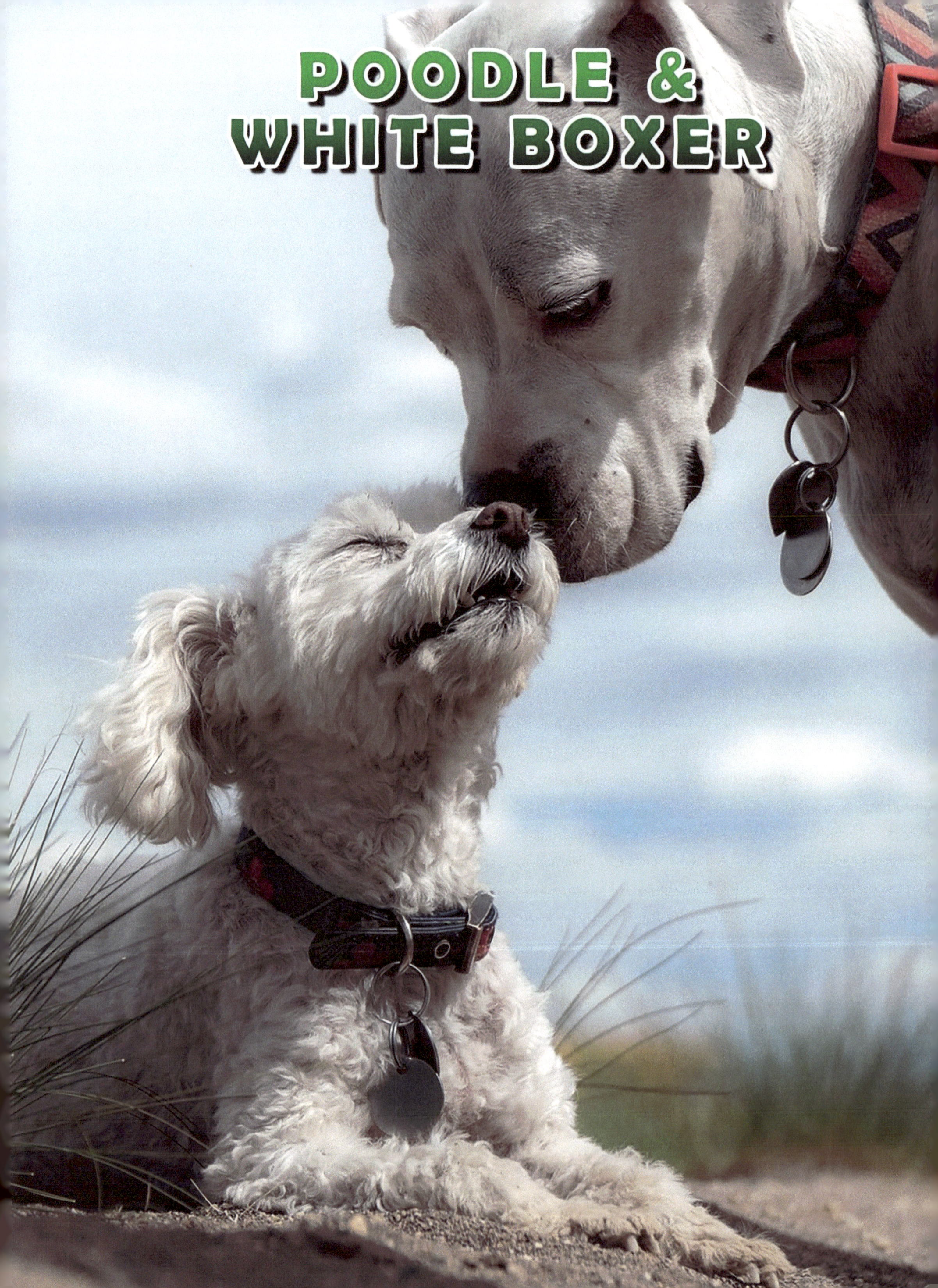

POODLE &
WHITE BOXER

PUG PUPPY

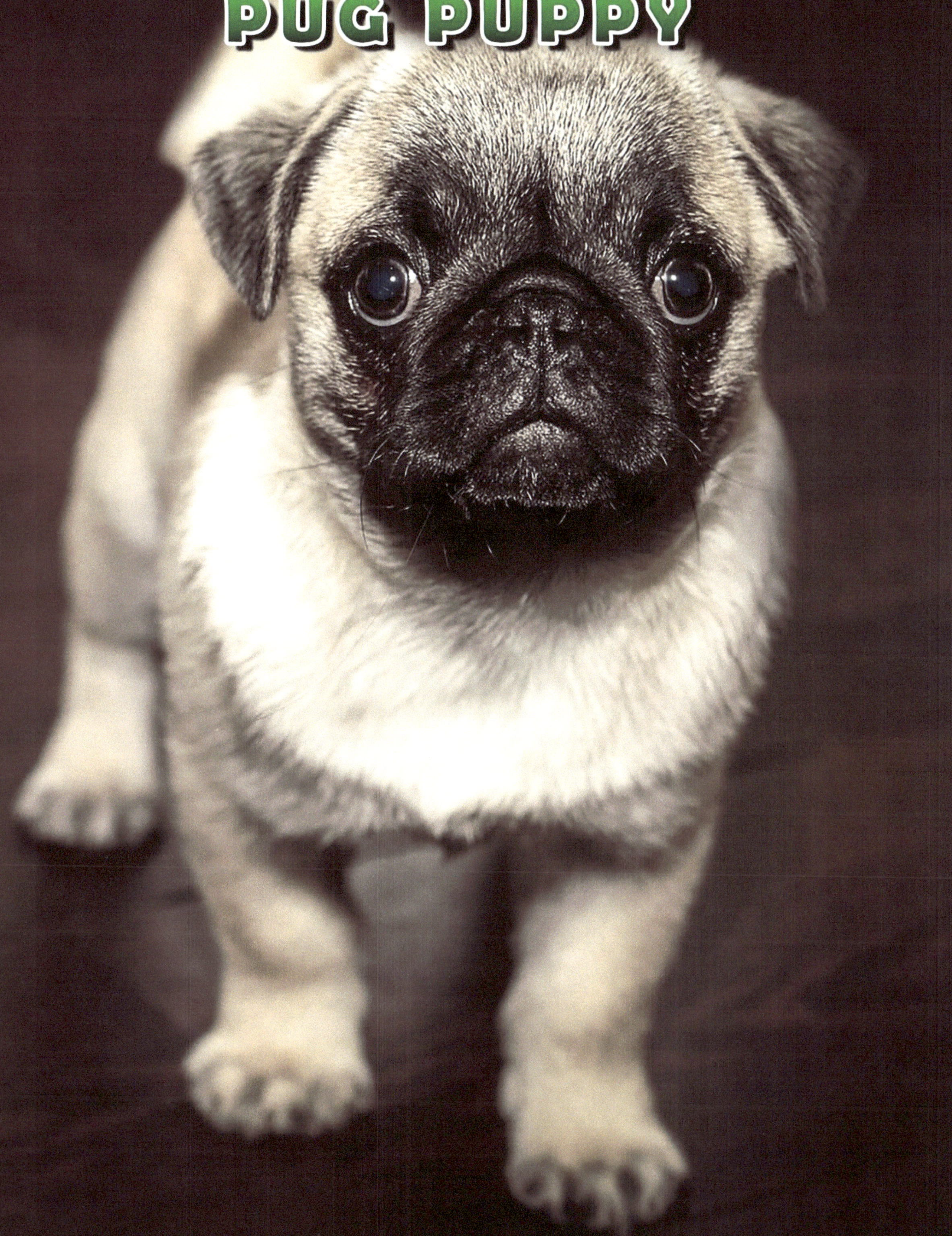

ROTTWEILER PUPPY

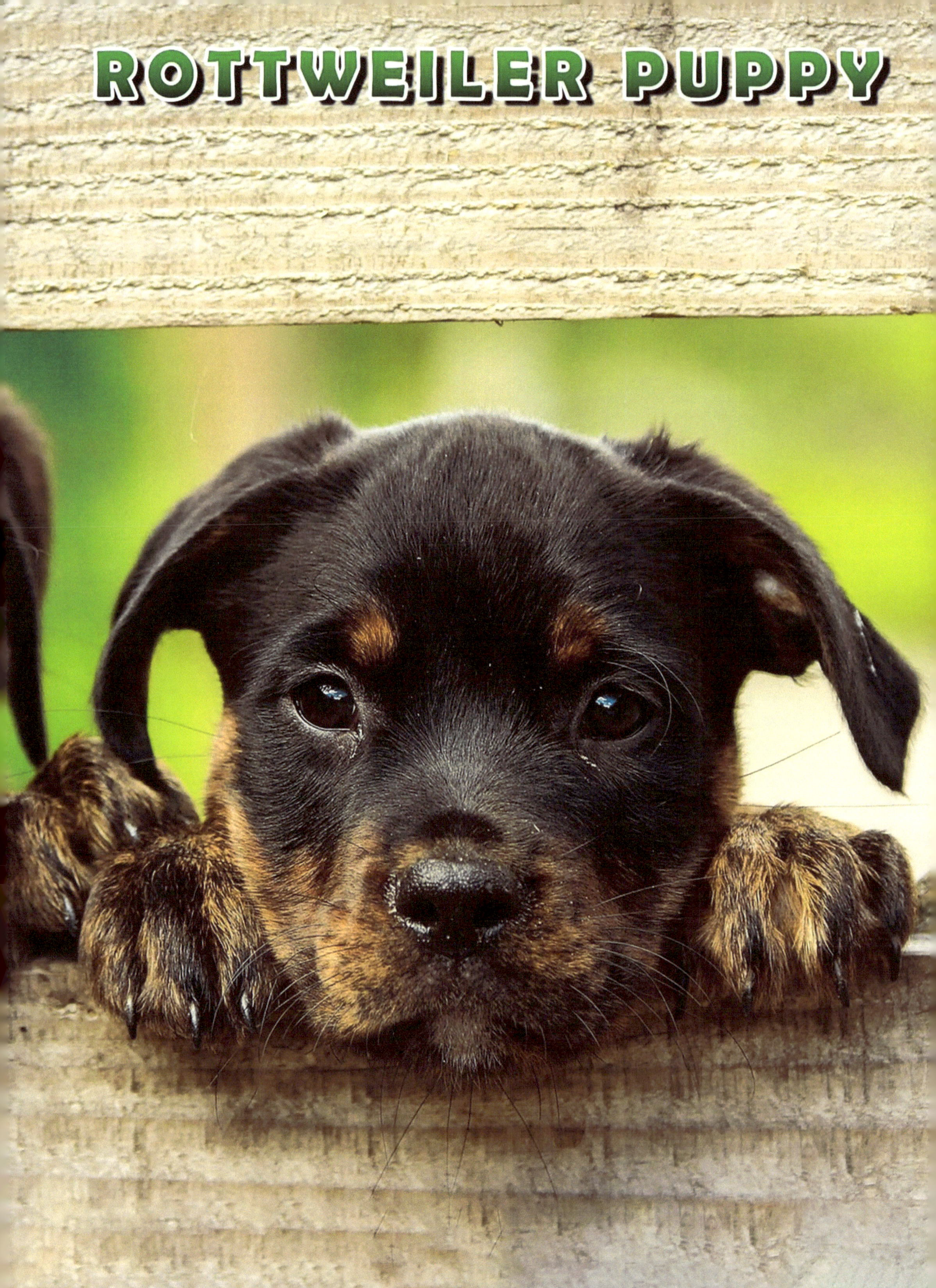

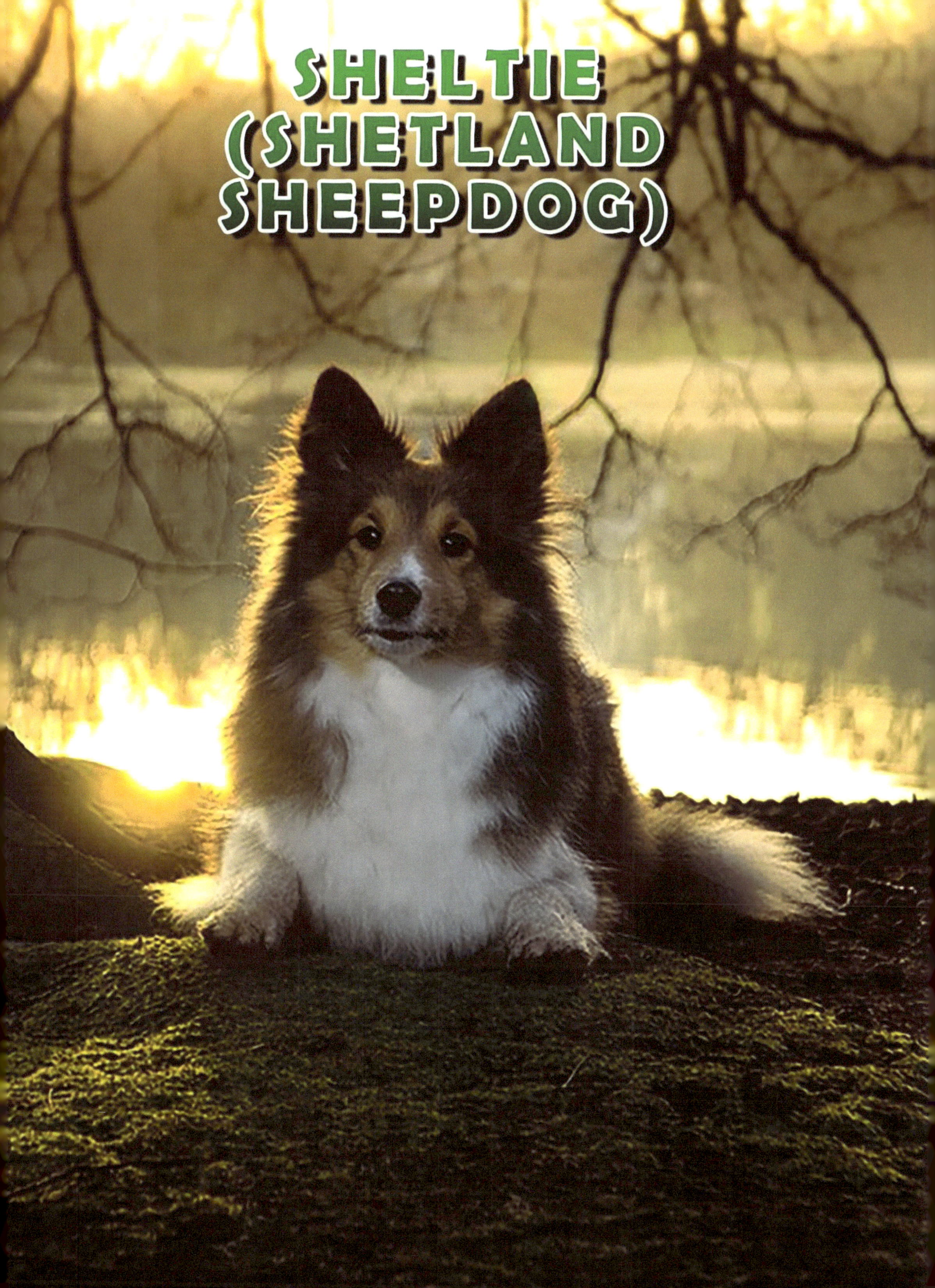
SHELTIE
(SHETLAND
SHEEPDOG)

SHIH TZU

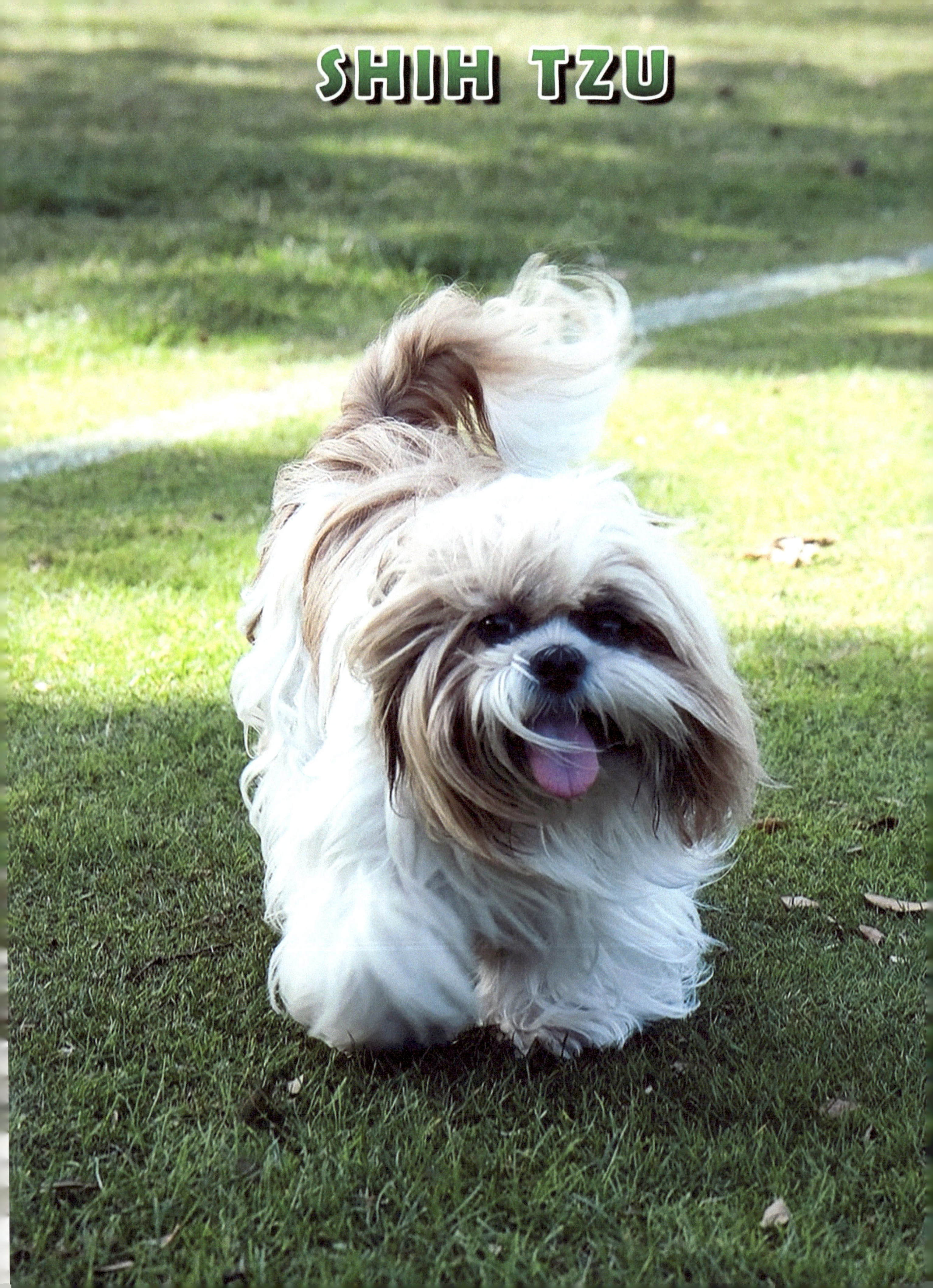

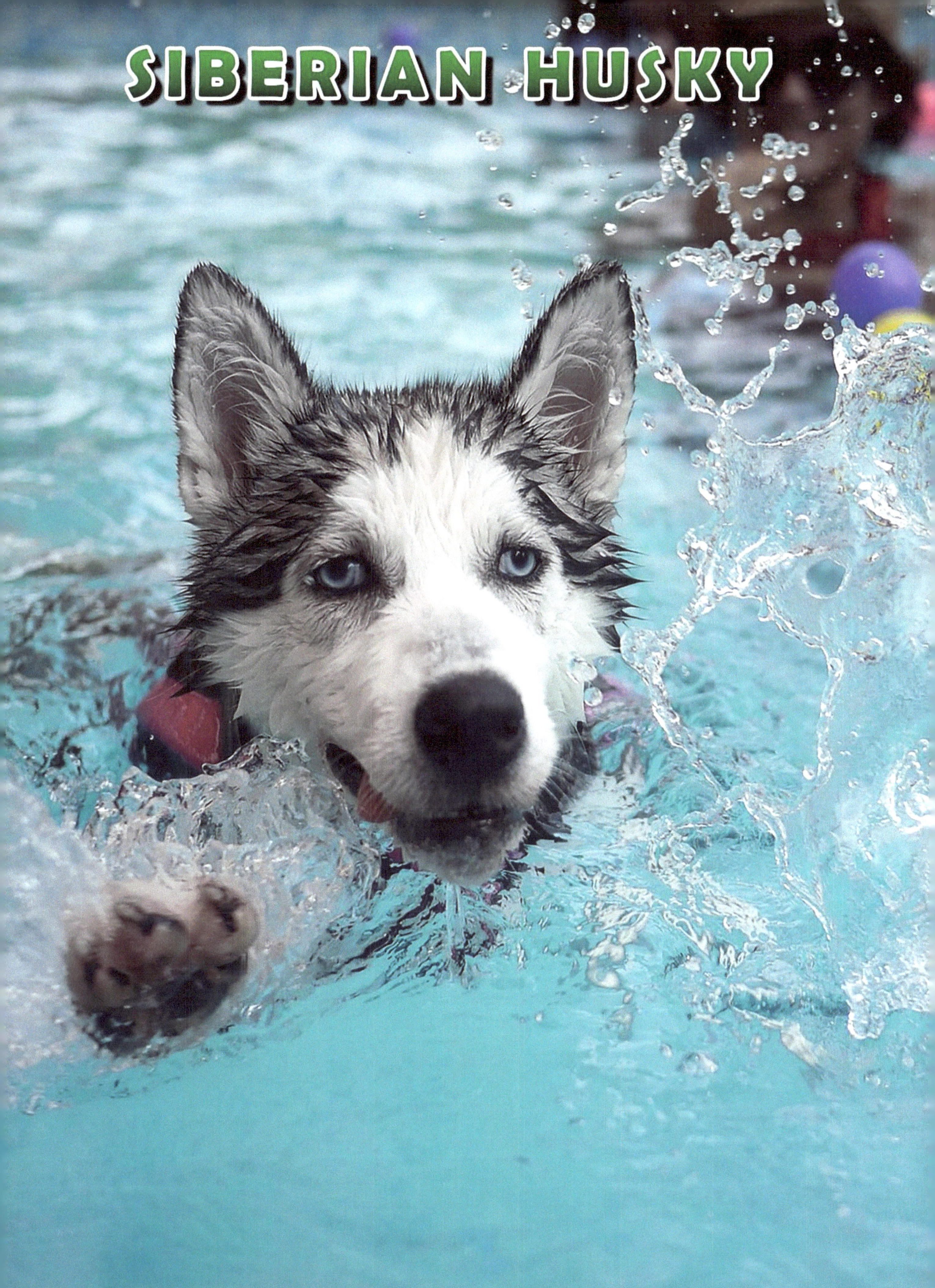

SIBERIAN HUSKY

ST. BERNARD

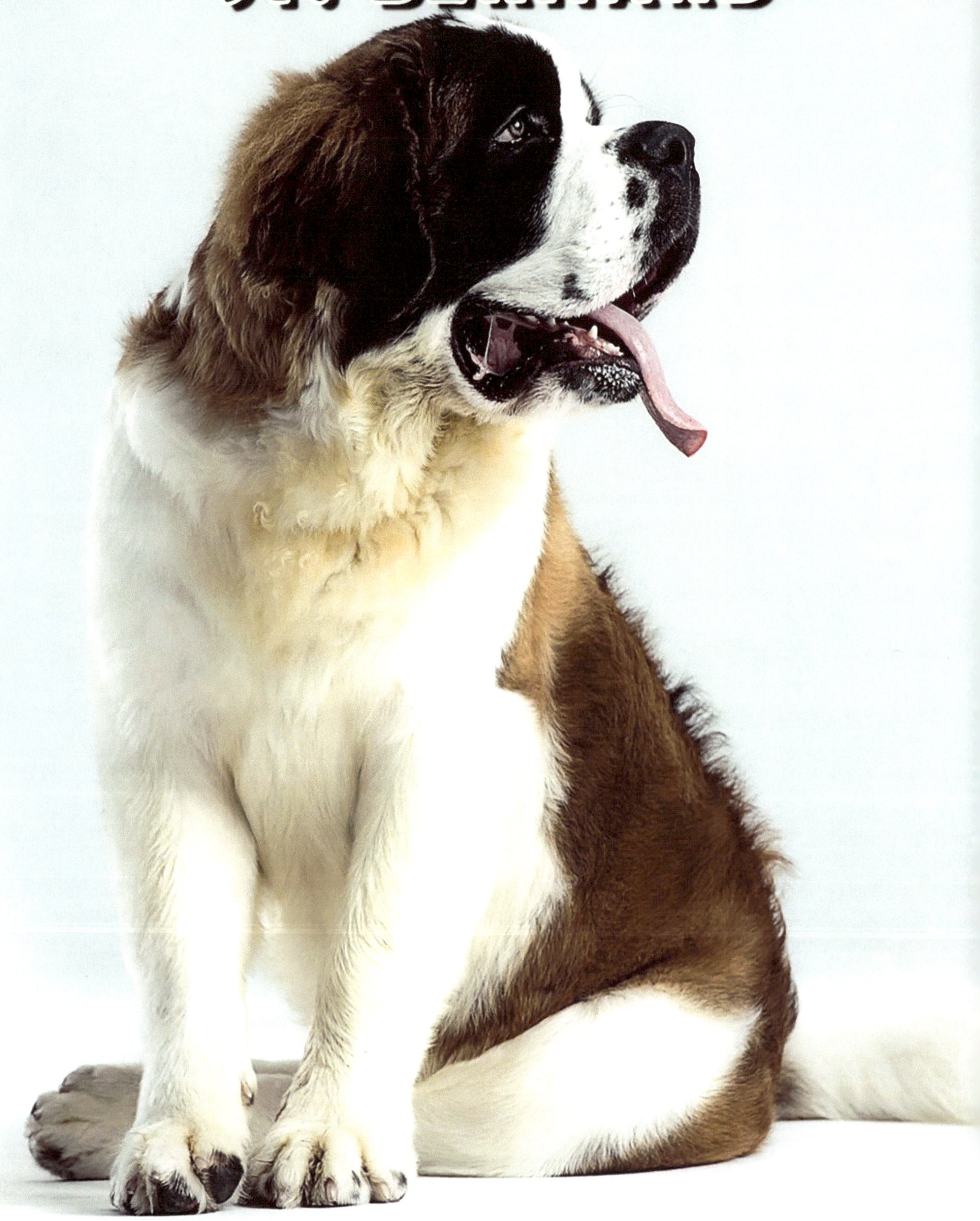

YORKSHIRE TERRIER

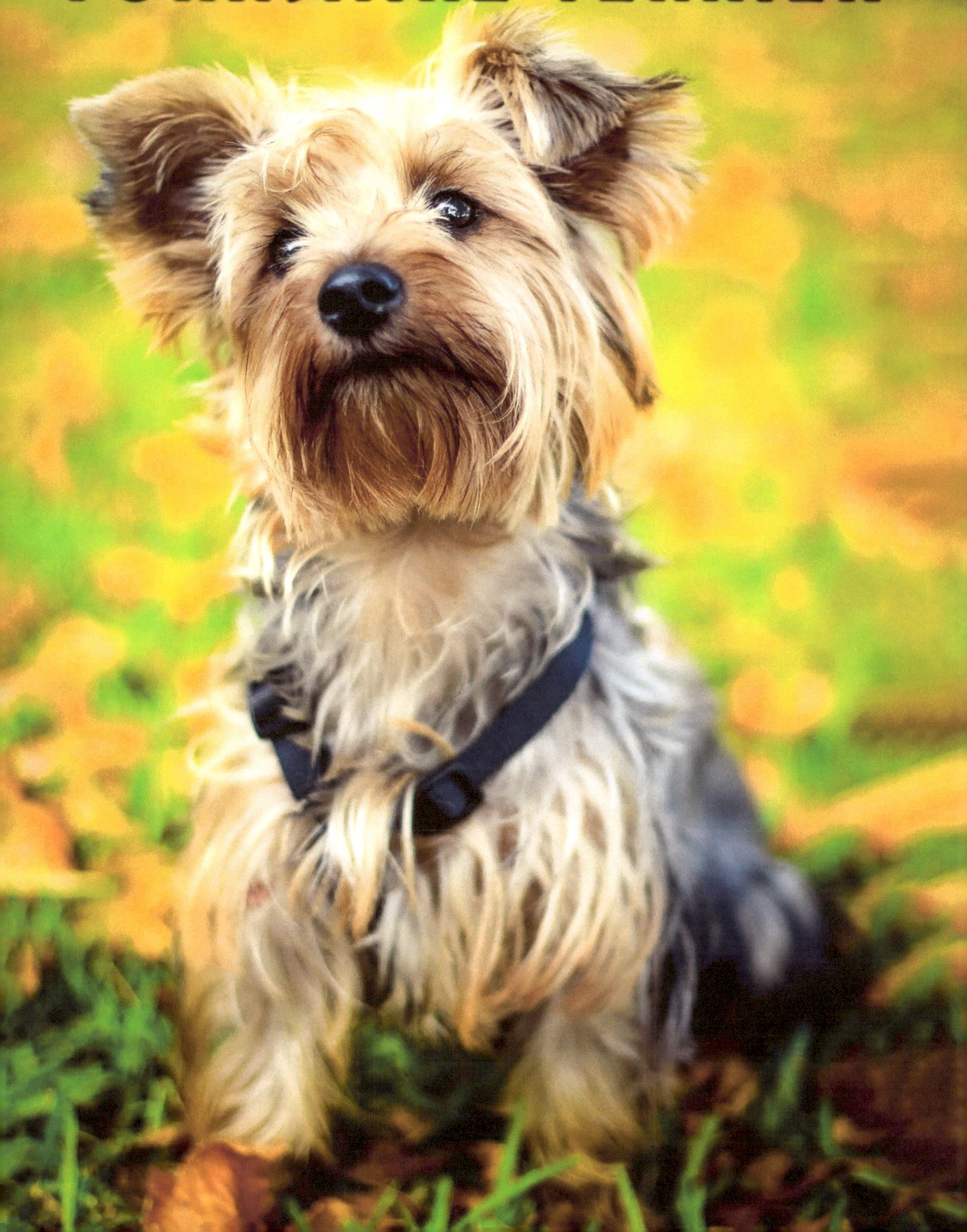

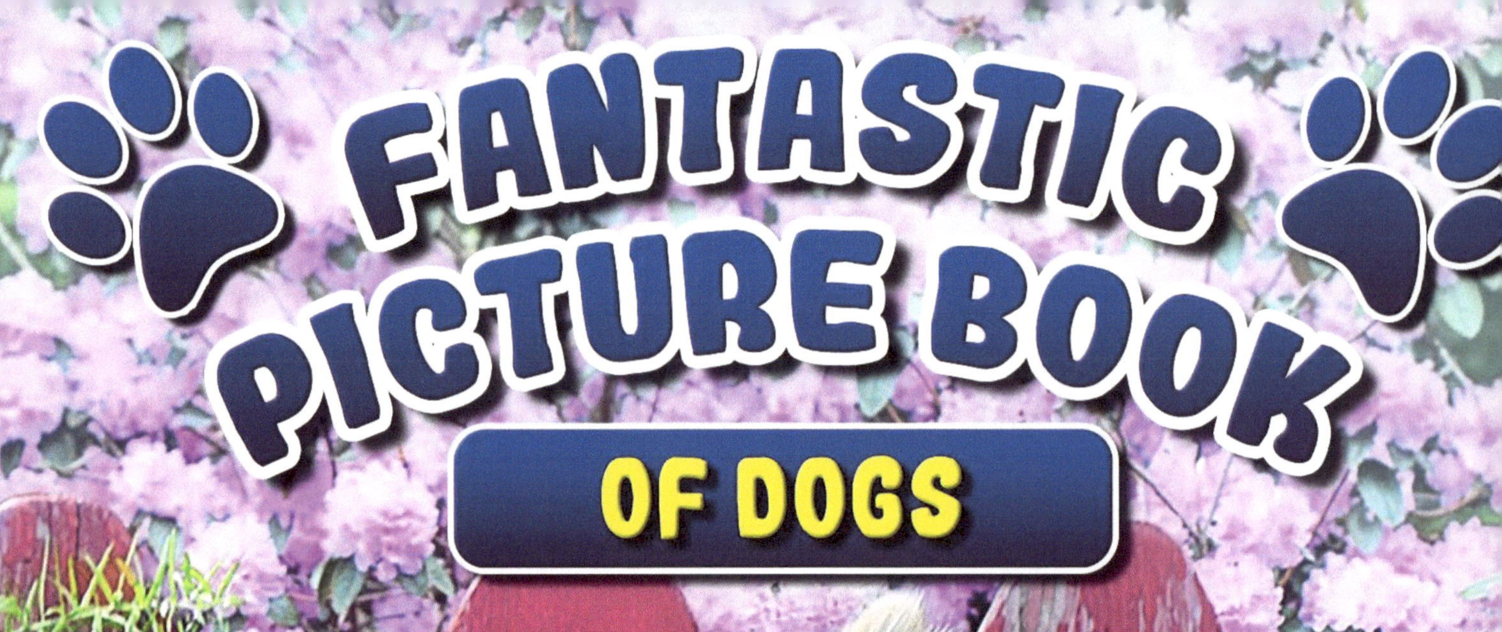

THANK YOU FOR BUYING.

If you have enjoyed this book, please tell your friends.

For more books, please visit:
etidbitz.com/books

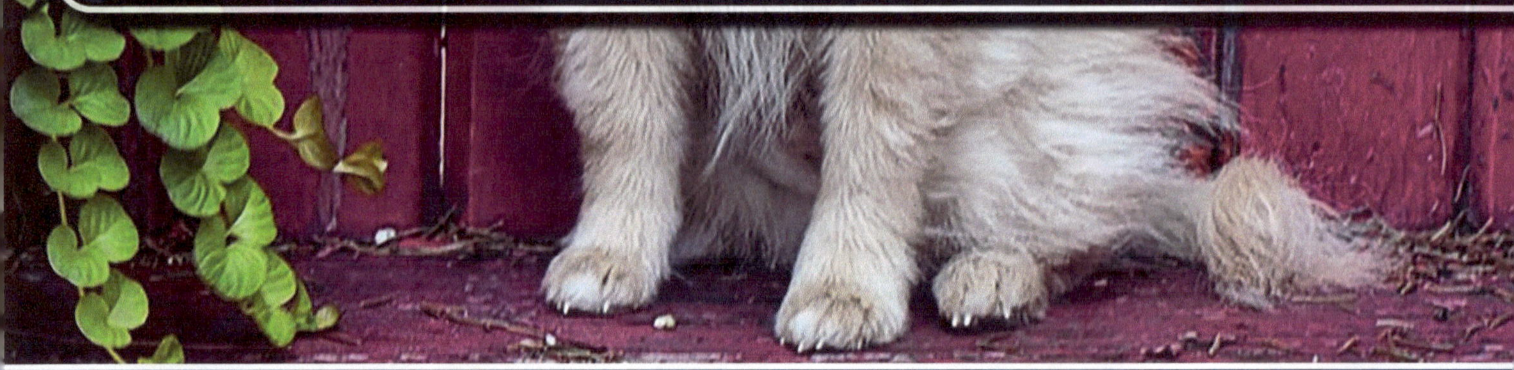